THE MARATHON METHOD

The 16-week Training Program That Prepares You
to Finish a Full or Half Marathon in Your Best Time

TOM HOLLAND
Foreword by Jeff Galloway

FAIR WINDS
PRESS

DEDICATION

This book is dedicated to my son Tommy. I look forward to running many miles and many marathons with you in the years to come.

Text © 2007 by Tom Holland

First published in the USA in 2007 by
Fair Winds Press, a member of
Quayside Publishing Group
33 Commercial Street
Gloucester, MA 01930

11 10 09 08 07   1 2 3 4 5

ISBN-13: 978-1-59233-259-5
ISBN-10: 1-59233-259-5

Library of Congress Cataloging-in-Publication Data available

Cover design by Poul Lange
Book design and layout by Leslie Haimes
Photography by Paul Johnson Photography (www.pauljohnsonphotography.com)

Printed and bound in USA

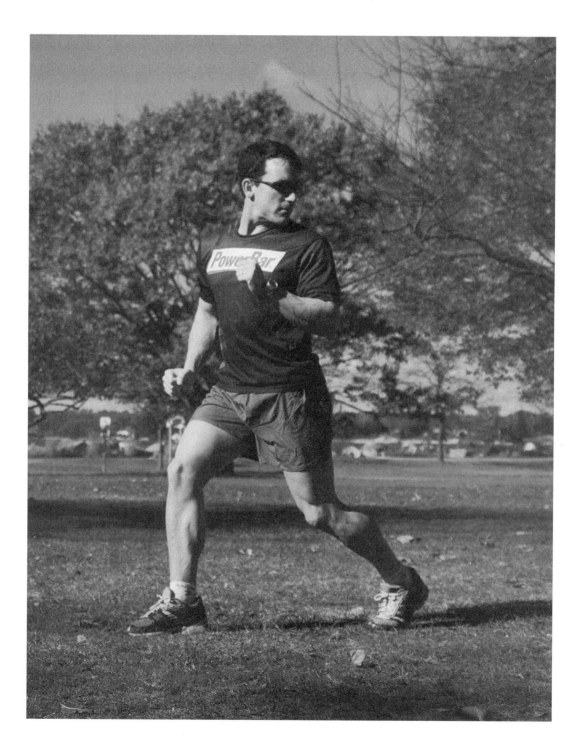

CONTENTS

FOREWORD

Today's marathoner is running against the lifestyle grain of society. While most citizens are becoming fatter and more sedentary, a growing number of former couch sitters have decided to test themselves by training for the most arduous event in the Olympic Games.

It seems that marathoners have always been perceived as different—and not always in a good way. In the early 1900s, journalists regularly warned potential Boston Marathon spectators that the event was so far beyond the capabilities of a "normal" human being that they might see someone die during the race. During the 1960s, when I started marathoning, there were other popular leisure-time addictions. Marathoners were often described as an eclectic mix of eccentrics. Since I was one, I'd have to admit that the description wasn't far off.

Today, there remain few significant challenges that must be done entirely by the individual. As I've listened to tens of thousands of people refer to the magic of crossing the finish line, I have heard extremely accomplished people say over and over again that completing a marathon is their most meaningful achievement. Others have related how the boost to body, mind, and spirit allowed them to change their lives in a positive direction.

Tom Holland has done a terrific job of bringing together the elements that can lead to marathon success. His advice comes from substantial experience and the lessons learned from making mistakes. If you absorb the information he offers and heed his advice, you may well avoid the problems that I hear about every day from participants in my running schools, retreats, and e-coaching practice. Tom and I agree that the marathon finish is entirely possible for most of us.

Having helped more than 100,000 marathoners reach their goals, I believe that marathon training doesn't have to hurt or result in injury. With the right ratio of running and walk breaks, virtually everyone can gain control over the training process and enjoy most or all of the activities that he or she would normally engage in.

Even after a steady increase in the number of marathoners over the past twenty years, finishing a 26.2-mile event puts you in an elite category—only one-tenth of 1 percent of the population completes a marathon each year.

You can do it!

Jeff Galloway
United States Olympian
www.JeffGalloway.com

Introduction

I come from a family of six boys, no girls, and I'm pretty sure my father took up running first and foremost to preserve what was left of his sanity. The amount of controlled chaos at home was probably directly proportional to the distances my father ran, so before long he was running marathons. Lots of them.

MY FIRST MARATHON

Like most runners, he would run longer on weekends, when he had more time. At the age of nine, I began to accompany him on his long slow distance or **LSD** runs, pedaling my little yellow bike with the banana seat alongside him as he put in the miles. We lived in a hilly town, and my dad would have to push me from behind to help me summit what seemed like unending peaks to my nine-year-old eyes and tiny quads. I'm sure that this was quality hill training for him and that he benefited from the added workload. He owes me.

When I was ten, my father entered me in my first organized race. Five kilometers, 3.1 miles . . . sheer heaven. We didn't run together, and I ran it like a Labrador that has been let out to run in a wide open field on a warm summer's day. No warm-up, no pacing, just off like a rocket. My father was waiting for me as I staggered across the finish line, all sweat and smiles. I accepted my wooden Popsicle stick with my finishing place written on it from the volunteer, and from that day forward I was hooked.

So I continued to run races with my father as the years went on, but as I grew older these shared experiences became less and less frequent. My dad kept running, but I became involved with other sports and girls (and not necessarily in that order). I attended Boston College and, although I still exercised, it was primarily for vanity's sake and not for health.

Boston is home to the prestigious Boston Marathon, which is scheduled on

Patriots' Day, a holiday in Massachusetts, and the entire state seems to turn out to cheer on the runners. For several years, I lived on Commonwealth Avenue, which is part of the marathon course, right after the infamous "Heartbreak Hill." We college kids would stand outside all day, swilling cheap beer and watching the runners swarm by, bragging about how we could all do it and placing bets on how we would absolutely do it the next year. This happened every April, but everyone had their excuses come January as to why he or she couldn't run that year.

My father continued to run marathons while I enjoyed college life. During my senior year, while home on Christmas break, he said he had a bib number for me and I could run the marathon with him if I so desired. This was a big deal, because the Boston Marathon is essentially by invitation only. You need to run a certain qualifying time based on your age in order to participate. (A chart with the current Boston Marathon qualifying times can be found on page 57.) A small number of people run as "bandits," unofficial runners who begin at the back of the pack and do not receive finisher medals or finishing times. Bandits are usually college kids, guys running dressed as Elvis or wearing Superman costumes, and others who just want to be a part of the race but fail to qualify.

So I took him up on the offer. I was going to run my first marathon in Boston that April.

Now you must realize that I had no plan, no coach, no training schedule, and no book like this to help tailor my preparation. I also had no clue what I was getting into. I was both naive and arrogant. I had seen the body types running by me down Commonwealth Avenue year after year, and most of them looked much more out of shape than I was. I could do this; no problem.

I did have my father, however. I had seen what he did to prepare for his marathons and had accompanied him on my bike for his longer workouts. I knew that I had to run a couple of times during the week and then run longer on the weekends. Occasionally, my dad would call me at school to check on my training.

"How's your training going? Did you get in some good runs this week?"

"Absolutely. I am right on track."

You would think that being raised Catholic, going to church every Sunday, and attending a Jesuit institution would prevent me from blatantly lying to my father about my training. You would be wrong.

I wasn't running at all.

Oh, I was still doing my push ups and sit ups. I was going to the gym and doing bicep's curls and tricep's press-downs. I wanted to look good, but I wasn't running.

And so my father kept checking in, and I continued to tell little white lies. I would have been well served by going to confession, admitting my lying ways to the priest, and receiving not a penance of several Hail Marys but an assignment of three short weekly runs and a long slow distance run every Sunday before church.

But the months flew by, and soon it was just three weeks until the marathon. I found myself at home for the weekend, so there could be no fibbing about my running, and I knew that I had better do something to prepare for the 26.2-mile journey I would soon undertake. Early one Sunday morning, I laced on my clunky cross-trainers (not running shoes), grabbed my enormous Walkman (this was 1991; no MP3 players), and set out on my first official long run. It was a beautiful day and, just like Forrest Gump, I kept running and running. I traveled up and down the hilly back roads of Connecticut with the music pumping through my headphones and my heart pumping from the workout. After roughly two hours of running with no particular route in mind, I found myself back at home, sweaty, sore, and spent. There. I was ready for Boston.

That was my first and last training run in preparation for the marathon. But don't assume that I did no preparation whatsoever: I spent several hours making a fantastic music mix chock full of big-haired '80s bands to power me along.

I spoke to my father the night before the race. Having seen me run in my cross-trainers at home, he asked if I had purchased real running shoes. I told him no, that I would be fine in what I had. He said something about bringing shoes for me, and we made plans to meet at a small church in Hopkinton at the race start.

Once again, my college apartment was right on the race course, mile twenty-one on Commonwealth Avenue. Police barricades lined the empty street as I jumped into a taxi on that Monday morning and told the driver to take me to the start of the Boston Marathon.

The Boston Marathon is a point-to-point race, which means that you do not start and finish in the same place. We were essentially driving the course backward as we sped down the highway. After driving for almost an hour, the gravity of the situation suddenly hit me like a ton of bricks:

Wait a minute. I had to run all the way.

And then five more miles . . .

Plus two-tenths.

This is not good.

At that instant, I had a moment of clarity and realized that I was in for a very, very long day of suffering. I was getting tired just riding in the taxi to the start; how the heck did I plan on running all the way back?

But the weather was spectacular as we arrived in the small town of Hopkinton amid throngs of bodies milling about. The pungent odor of Bengay hung in the air as runners stretched against signposts, lay sprawled on the ground on old newspapers, applied homemade ointments to unmentionable areas, and peed in the bushes. And peed in the trees, bushes, fences, and against houses. There was an awful lot of peeing going on.

I wound my way through the narrow streets to find the small white church and my father waiting next to it. He was holding a pair of running shoes for me, which I grudgingly accepted. He tried to give me last-minute advice, but his words faded as my mind wandered and my stomach churned. The feeling of energy and excitement generated by the thousands of runners was infectious, unlike any feeling I had ever experienced. There was a tension in the air, albeit a uniquely positive one. The looks on the faces around me were of controlled anticipation, like a child on Christmas morning right

before his parents say he can go downstairs and open the presents.

My father and I had different bib numbers—mine was a much lower number than his. This meant that I would start in a corral ahead of him and cross the start line ten or fifteen minutes before he did. I remained cocky until the very end: As he gave me his final words of marathon wisdom, I bid him adieu and said that I would meet him at the finish line.

Much like a cow being herded into a corral or pen, you line up in a certain area usually designated by your bib number. Some races assign corrals by asking you your estimated finishing time on your application. Be honest and realistic when answering; you will not enjoy running with a group that is too fast or too slow.

If you want to run with a friend and you are not in the same corral, some races will allow you to move backward but not forward. In other words, the runner with the "faster" number (usually a lower number) may be allowed to join the "slower" corral, but not vice versa. Ask a volunteer whether this is allowed if you wish to do so.

I trailed the throngs of runners siphoning down the side streets to our corrals. I found the corral that corresponded to my bib number and filed in, packed shoulder to shoulder like sardines with runners who didn't smell much better.

The strains of our national anthem wafted through the midday air and fighter planes buzzed overhead as we shifted our feet in nervous anticipation of the start. I rewound my tape and put on my headphones. The opening guitar chords of Living Colour's "Cult of Personality" filled my head as the loud report of a cannon pierced the air. We were off.

Fifteen thousand people attempting to move quickly through the narrow suburban streets of Hopkinton is quite a sight. You can't really start running for some time, because the runners need to funnel ahead of you in one enormous mass of bodies. You run five steps, walk for three, jog for two, and the progression continues for several long minutes.

But soon enough, I was running. The weather was warm and the April sky was crystal clear; it was a perfect day for my first marathon attempt. Throngs of people lined both sides of the street: Little kids held out orange slices, families lounged in beach chairs, and people waved homemade signs offering encouragement to their loved ones. As we climbed our first hill, the theme song from *Rocky*, the "Eye of the Tiger," blasted from a driveway on our right. I was on top

of the world; this was going to be a piece of cake.

I had no idea what pace I was running, but in hindsight, it was definitely way too fast. Runners are renowned for starting races like Labrador retrievers chasing a squirrel, especially newbie (and naive) runners like I was then. You get swept up in the electric energy of the moment and it's extremely difficult to hold back. This is especially deadly when facing a marathon distance— you will pay dearly later in the race for a lack of pacing.

On I sprinted, the marathon mix pounding through my headphones and blending with the cheers from the crowds. I flew through Ashland and hammered through Framingham. The temperature was rising and the gray cotton Boston College T-shirt I was wearing was soaked with sweat and clinging to my body. As I approached mile ten and the town of Natick, something unexpected happened.

I hit the "Wall."

Better yet, I crashed, smashed, and plowed into the Wall. Hard. Headfirst and at full speed.

The Wall is a term used to describe the point in an endurance race when your body says, "No more." I believe the two causes of hitting the Wall are a lack of proper training and a failure to ingest proper amounts of carbohydrates before and during the race. If you train correctly, as I will later explain in full detail, you will never have to experience the Wall. Back then I did not come remotely close to training correctly. Hitting the Wall usually happens to runners at around mile twenty. But even people who undertrain usually practice with long runs of at least sixteen or eighteen miles before taking on a marathon. Not one run of twelve miles, as I had.

Needless to say, I thought I was dying. My legs felt like lead and a severe fog had settled on my brain. I slowed to a sluggish crawl, stripped off my sweat-soaked shirt and tucked it into my shorts. My Walkman had turned into a twenty-pound dumbbell and I needed to get rid of it. I spotted a young boy standing on the side of the road and did my best Mean Joe Green in the Coke commercial:

"Hey kid, catch."

I tossed him my Walkman as he stared at me in confusion and wonder before tearing off into his house with his new acquisition. I'm pretty sure he came to the marathon the following year expecting more freebies from the runners.

I continued to stumble down the road as cramps invaded my quads. I wasn't even at the halfway point and I was finished. And just when I thought it was all over, I felt a tap on my shoulder.

It was my dad.

I didn't know at the time how beaten up I looked, but he could tell I was hurting. He asked how I was doing and I told him my legs were two enormous cramps. We were approaching a medical tent and he disappeared inside. He emerged with some strange gel on a stick and told me to rub it into my legs. Believing that this was some kind of prescription cramp eliminator, I did as I was told. Sure enough, my legs felt a little better and we made our way back to the race. Months later, my dad admitted that the miracle salve was plain old Vaseline. It was one of my first experiences with the powerful "placebo effect," a phenomenon by which something works simply because you believe or expect it to work, regardless of the actual ingredients. It is a striking example of the awesome power the mind has over the body.

Miles twelve through nineteen were a blur. I plodded along while my dad used every trick to take my mind off the pain. I don't even remember running up the grueling Heartbreak Hill. I do remember emerging from my brain fog as we passed the drunken crowds at Boston College and approached my apartment.

"Why don't we go inside?" I heard my dad say over the screaming undergraduates. "You can take a shower and then finish the race."

"No way. If we stop now, I'm never starting up again. Let's finish this."

And on we went. Before too long, the famous CITGO sign appeared in the distance. I knew that that was a good sign (pun intended); it meant the finish line was within reach. As we rounded the final turn and I saw the finish line, I was flooded with emotion, a sensation I will never forget. It is a feeling that I experience every time I finish a marathon, an ultramarathon (any running race over 26.2 miles is considered an ultramarathon), or an Ironman. It's the reason that more than 60,000 people try to get in to the New York City Marathon every year. There is an incredible sense of accomplishment that comes from tackling something that challenges your mind and your body. Sigmund Freud postulated that we avoid pain and seek out pleasure. I contend that true happiness and fulfillment come from seeking pleasure through pain. Not injury-causing pain, but pain in the sense that your will is put to the test. You undertake something extremely difficult, entirely of your own choosing. You invest large amounts of physical and emotional energy based on faith and the belief that you can achieve something that is far from guaranteed. And the more you invest, the more obtainable your goals and the more incredible the pleasure that waits for you on the other side of that finish line.

Crossing the finish line with my dad back in 1991 was a pivotal point in my life, one that I look back upon often. Since then, I have run more than twenty marathons, three ultramarathons, and twelve Ironman triathlons. I have qualified for and run the Boston race seven years in a row, beginning in 2000. That first marathon took me four and a half hours to complete; now my best time is under three hours. Running has become a lifestyle, a healthy addiction, a part of my job, and a way of life.

If this is your first marathon, I envy you. Although all finishes are memorable, there is nothing like your first. Be prepared for a life-changing experience. If you have run more then one marathon and have turned to this book for further guidance, I can make you faster and less prone to injury while having more fun—and all in just sixteen weeks. Four months is all I ask of you. I guarantee that if you follow my training plans and implement my proven strategies and techniques, you will not be disappointed.

What is this book about? It contains all of the information I desperately needed before my first marathon: training plans, plus tips on nutrition, hydration, gear, pacing, the mental training, injury prevention, strength training, flexibility, and much more. You will learn from my mistakes so that you can avoid making them yourself. You will learn from my experience and those of my clients so that you can have the best marathon experience possible. If you finish your race with a smile on your face and, once the soreness has subsided, start searching for another race to train for, then I have done my job successfully.

NOTE: Although this book deals with training for both a half marathon and a full marathon, the term marathon will be used throughout. The vast majority of concepts apply to both distances and those that do not will be covered separately.

CHAPTER 1
Why Run?

This is a simple question that I am asked all the time. Why do you run? Allow me to list a few of the positive side effects of cardiovascular exercise, specifically running, which include the following:

1. Increases HDL levels (the "good cholesterol")

2. Helps prevent and control diabetes

3. Lowers blood pressure

4. Increases cardiovascular function

5. Promotes weight loss

6. Helps prevent cardiovascular disease

7. Increases insulin sensitivity (decreased insulin sensitivity can lead to type II diabetes)

8. Increases bone mineral density

9. Increases self-confidence and self-esteem

10. Decreases symptoms of depression

This is by no means a comprehensive list. I always say that I run "for my head" first. Running provides me with a means to rid myself of stress. It is my "moving meditation." No matter how I feel beforehand, I always feel dramatically better after a run. Running is simple. It costs almost nothing. You can do it almost anywhere. You can run alone or with friends. Simply put: Running makes you look better, feel better, and live longer, all at the same time.

That's pretty darn good.

The question should really be, "Why don't you run?" Open almost any magazine and you'll be bombarded with full-page ads from big pharmaceutical companies advertising their newest drugs—drugs that more often than not medicate conditions that can be greatly improved just by running. Having trouble sleeping? Cardiovascular exercise has been proven to help. Need to improve your blood-lipid profile? Running is excellent for that, too. This is not to say that we don't need medicine, but we might benefit from less pharmacological intervention and more running.

Then there are television ads pitching the latest drugs, and it's difficult to determine what they are even intended to cure. These commercials always end with the same line, "Ask your doctor about Willfixya." How about a few ads that say, "Ask your doctor about exercise"?

We runners know the constant cry of non-runners all too well. They proclaim that "running is bad for your knees." Unfortunately, many doctors expound this falsehood to their patients, but they must not be reading the research on this subject. There is actually little scientific support for the claim that running causes arthritis, and several studies suggest just the opposite. Stanford University began a continuing study in 1984 in which 500 middle-aged runners from a running club were followed for twenty years. When they were compared to a group of non-runners, the runners did not have higher rates of arthritis, and they appeared to have a lower risk of muscle- and skeletal-related disability and pain.

Another study conducted by the Cooper Institute and the Centers for Disease Control and Prevention found no correlation between running and arthritis of the hip or knee. Finally, in a study that compared runners with swimmers, the runners were less likely to require surgery for arthritis or to have severe pain in the hips and knees.

Now if you've had an acute injury to the knee or a specific biomechanical issue, running may indeed exacerbate the condition. It has been my experience, however, that the vast majority of these cases can be remedied through strength training, flexibility training, and intelligent **periodization**.

Periodization: The gradual cycling of specificity, intensity, and volume to achieve peak levels of fitness while preventing injury and burnout, often for a specific event. For runners, the major use of periodization is the systematic increasing and decreasing of weekly running mileage.

I contend that running is crucial to our overall well-being because it so clearly illuminates our weak links, showing us what we need to work on to be as balanced and as strong as possible. Running is a test of sorts. We engage in this test and learn quickly what we as individuals must focus on in our overall fitness program. If a client begins a running program and after a period of time experiences lower back pain, should he stop and assume that the running is the culprit? Or should he perhaps question why his

Jim Fixx: Setting the Record Straight

Jim Fixx was the man credited with bringing about the jogging and running explosion of the late '70s. In 1977, he published The Complete Book of Running, which sold more than a million copies, spent eleven weeks at number one on the best-seller list, and was an inspiration to millions. In 1980, he published Jim Fixx's Second Book of Running as a follow-up.

Unfortunately, Fixx died from a massive heart attack during his daily run at the age of fifty-two. Many non-runners and comedians alike have used him as an example of why they don't run or why running is a complete waste of time. Once you learn the facts about him, however, you realize how specious and uninformed their argument is.

Here's the truth about Jim Fixx: Had he not taken up running at the age of thirty-five, he probably would not have lived much longer. He weighed 214 pounds and smoked two packs of cigarettes a day. Years later, after he started running regularly, he weighed less than 160 pounds and had quit smoking. Family history is an enormous risk factor when it comes to heart disease: Fixx's father suffered a heart attack at the age of thirty-five and subsequently died from another at forty-two.

Dr. Mary McQuillen, the doctor who performed the autopsy on Fixx, reported that the blockages in his arteries were such that he would have died many years earlier had his heart not been strengthened as a result of running.

back hurts and examine ways to fix it? Does he have weak spinal erectors? Are his hamstrings tight? Are his abdominal muscles weak? If he were simply to stop running and ignore his lower back pain, it would inevitably resurface and probably in a much more serious incident. This is what I love about running. Through running we can learn so much about our bodies and become stronger as a result, not weaker through injury.

If you are like so many millions trying to lose weight, then running is among the fastest, cheapest, and easiest ways to shed pounds and keep them off. Once again, I spend the majority of my time running with my private clients. We engage in strength training, but it is often as a means to fix the imbalances and weaknesses exposed through running. Sure, I could give clients all the fancy exercises pictured in magazines and trendy workouts with the newest equipment, but that wouldn't get us to our goals of weight loss, overall muscle tone, and optimal physical health. Weight loss is actually a very basic concept made much more confusing by unqualified people trying to make a quick buck. It's all about energy in and energy out. Take in more than you burn each day and you will gain weight. Expend more than you consume each day and you will lose weight. As far as which exercise is a top calorie burner, or one of the best ways to achieve "negative daily energy balance," that's easy. It's running.

So there you have it. We run for our head, we run for our health, and we run for our vanity. We run to push our limits and to challenge who we are. We become both mentally and physically stronger with each mile and with each new goal attained.

More than 60,000 people applied for one of the 30,000 spots in the New York City Marathon last year. No one is making these people run; there must be some kind of substantial payoff.

FAITH AND TRUST

By buying this book and following my training plans and advice, you are essentially hiring me as your running coach. I want to thank you. I have found nothing more satisfying than helping others push their boundaries and achieve goals that they hadn't dreamed were possible. There is also nothing quite like assisting someone in identifying a goal, working hard toward it, and ultimately achieving it. Over the years, I have trained numerous clients to run their first marathon and then ran the race with them, pacing them through to the finish line. Each of these experiences has been incredible. By taking me on as your coach, you are putting a great deal of faith and trust in me. Training for a marathon is a commitment of time and money, and you don't want to waste either one. You have faith that what is in this book will help you achieve your goals, and you trust that I possess the knowledge, experience, and passion necessary to warrant following my advice. To have this necessary faith and trust, you should know who your coach is and what he is all about, so let me tell you about my knowledge, experience, and passion.

I received my undergraduate degree from Boston College in communications and a master's degree in exercise science with a concentration in sports psychology from Southern Connecticut State University. I am certified by the American College of Sports Medicine, the National Strength and Conditioning Association, the National Academy of Sports Medicine, and the American Council on Exercise.

I worked as a personal trainer and group fitness instructor for years at such clubs as Reebok, Equinox, New York Sports Clubs, and Crunch. I have worked with more than a thousand clients from all walks of life: old, young, out of shape, and elite athlete. I have designed programs and trained clients to run 5Ks through ultramarathons, Ironman triathlons, and more. One of my favorite races was when I trained and paced a seventy-five-year-old female client to "run" her first 5K in Central Park.

As my business evolved, I began to focus more on writing, videos, lectures, and camps, as well as training a small clientele one-on-one and online. Now, I primarily run with my private clientele. The day starts early, and some days I log thirty miles with clients by 10 a.m. People often say to my clients, "You pay somebody to run with you?" Yes, and they get an enormous amount from these sessions. Many clients have a weight loss goal, and what better way to achieve this than by running? And as we run, we discuss nutrition, hydration, pacing, form, clothing—everything that is covered in this book. We also set race goals, and we achieve them. Most important, when an ache or a pain arises, I am right there and can react quickly to diagnose and deal with it. All of these experiences have put me in a unique position to learn firsthand from hundreds of real-life "experiments."

Finally, I have been running my whole life, from those early training runs and races with my dad to today. I have run marathons all over the world, including nine in Boston (seven consecutively); three in New York; two in San Diego; one each in Philadelphia, Chicago, Westchester, Miami, Big Sur, Hartford, Las Vegas, Honolulu, Rome, and Dublin; and the Marine Corps Marathon. I have experienced what running at a high altitude can do during my thirty-six-mile "Run to the Sun" ultramarathon on Maui. It is billed as the only point-to-point marathon where you can see the finish from the start line, and we ran from sea level up to the 10,023-foot summit of Mount Haleakala (I finished ninth). I learned more about going long as well as trail running during the JFK fifty-miler in Maryland, which I also ran with a client. I have also competed in twelve Ironman triathlons, consisting of a 2.4-mile swim, a 112-mile bike ride, and a marathon run. Plus, I have completed hundreds of 5Ks, 10Ks, and half marathons.

And most important? I am injury free. But much more on that later.

MY COACHING PHILOSOPHY

Before we get started, you need to know about my coaching philosophy. It breaks down into two simple points:

1. *My Goal Is to Get You to the Start Line Injury Free:* It is so easy for a personal trainer to tell a client to do 100 push ups, 50 squats, or 200 crunches. Likewise, it would be easy for me to create training plans with a ridiculous amount of training volume and be known as that "really tough coach." That's a no-brainer. There are plenty of coaches like that out there, with plenty of overtrained and injured clients. When a client becomes injured, the blame is often expressed in one of two ways. First, the coach will tell the client that he or she did not work hard enough and that caused the injury. Second, the client comes to believe that he or she cannot run because of some genetic weakness. Either way, clients blame themselves. Of course, if the client does not adhere to the coach's training plan and does too much of one thing and not enough of another, then he or she should accept some responsibility. But if they follow the coach's advice and still fall short, often repeatedly, then the coach's methodology has to be called into question.

What's difficult as a coach is providing the least amount of training to accomplish the greatest goal. "Train less, run your best!" As an exercise physiologist, I am always looking for the safest way to achieve the greatest results in the least amount of time when it comes to fitness. There is no honor in getting injured as a result of running too much. The ultimate goal is to be healthy and running into our seventies, eighties, and beyond. Why wouldn't all coaches want this? I believe there are two reasons: lack of knowledge and ego. Some coaches do not have a firm grasp of exercise science, human physiology, biomechanics, and kinesiology and risk training their clients too hard. Others want to establish a reputation as a "tough" coach and deliberately push their runners too hard.

You must also realize that being injury free does not mean that issues will not present themselves. Of course they will. We all experience aches and pains, but the difference lies in how we deal with them. We do not "run through" pain that will eventually cause injury. We discover what the cause is and we fix it. We also behave proactively to prevent aches and pains from arising at all.

It is true that a significant percentage

of the runners at the starting line of a marathon are nursing training injuries. My first and foremost goal is to get you there injury free. It is much better to be 5 percent undertrained than 1 percent overtrained when it comes to an endurance race.

2. *You Can Have a Great Time and Run a Great Time:* In other words, race performance and race enjoyment are not mutually exclusive. The conventional wisdom is that if you are working really hard, you have to "wear" that pain—you have to look as if you are in serious agony. I completely disagree. One of my running secrets is to keep a smile on my face throughout the race. The faster I run and the more uncomfortable I feel, the bigger my smile. Frowning and negative thoughts create tension in the body. Tension affects you mentally as well as physiologically and will ultimately impair your performance. Is it easy to smile through the discomfort? Not at first, but when you make it part of your race strategy, you will be amazed at the results. I will discuss this much further in the section on mental training.

DOING VS. TEACHING

It may sound strange, but my goal in this book is not to teach you or to have you learn—it is simply to give you a plan for what to do. My focus is not to turn you into an exercise physiologist with a deep knowledge of the body's energy systems, biomechanics, or heart-rate responses.

To be honest, there are an infinite number of books and magazines that try to do that, and in my opinion, they only serve to make the author sound authoritative but have little relevance to the overwhelming majority of runners. Do you really need to know what your VO2 max is? Should I really enter into the debate over active isolated stretching versus passive stretching?

If your eyes are beginning to glaze over, do not fear, because that's not what my book is about. I treat you like one of my clients who has come to me with questions and is seeking advice.

I may not tell you about mitochondrial density and Type IIB muscle fibers, but I will discuss what you should eat during your training as well as what I personally eat. To run a marathon, do you need to understand the intricacies of the body's various energy systems? No, but you need to run. You need to strength train. You need to stretch, hydrate, fuel, and refuel properly, and you need to do all of these things consistently. You need to know the little tips and tricks that may seem insignificant but can make all the difference in your marathon experience. I will explain certain concepts when I feel it is necessary, but I want you to read this book and do what is required so you can have the best marathon experience possible. That doesn't mean doing more; it means focusing on what matters and what will deliver positive results. Yes, you can train less and run your best.

GOING LONG

I have met many people who have tried running, hated it, and quit. These people averaged around two- to three-mile runs and rarely ran much farther. I remember when I first started running—it was really hard for me as well! I didn't sprint out of the womb and run my first ultramarathon. In fact, I spent most of my high-school sports career injured with debilitating shin splints. If you were to tell me back then that I would be running ultramarathons later in life, I would have said you were experiencing some kind of runner's high.

When most people first engage in a running program, it is work. This holds true of any exercise program, but especially running, because it is difficult.

When people first begin to run, their breathing is labored, they may experience painful "side stitches," and they often feel like they are running ridiculously slowly. Afterward, they may have sore muscles, major fatigue, and chafing in places where they never knew rubbing even occurred. No wonder so many people quit! When I tell first-time runners that this is a normal response and that experienced runners felt just as lousy when they first started, they rarely believe me. They blame themselves, believing that they are just too unfit and that they will never be able to run and enjoy it.

I believe in what I call the "cardiovascular turning point," or CTP, a physiological state that occurs after running for a certain amount of time during each workout. It is not to be confused with the "runner's high" that comes after running for long periods of time; it is an initial point at which running begins to feel comfortable. It is a warm-up of sorts, and those who only run short distances may never experience this CTP. These are the same people who tend to quit running because it never becomes enjoyable for them.

I have found that most people experience this phenomenon once they've been running for between thirty and forty minutes. This is purely anecdotal, mind you;

CHAPTER 2
Setting Goals

I cannot overemphasize the importance of setting goals and setting the right ones. Without a goal to reach for, you have no real direction or plan. I do not begin to work with a client until we have first established our concrete goals and written them down. This is why setting the goal of completing a race is such a powerful one. It immediately fits two of the major criteria of effective goal setting: It is concrete and there is a definitive date of completion, namely race day.

PLANNING FOR GOALS

For many clients who come to me to lose weight and get in shape, I try to steer them toward a race goal as part of their program. Maybe a 5K to start, then a 10K, and so on. It provides focus and quantifiable results and demands the consistency of a set plan of action. Even though we might not discuss the possibility of running a marathon, I have to admit that it is always in the back of my mind.

Let me give you an example of goal setting with a client who contacted me several years ago. She was the head of a major company and worked insane hours—in other words, a textbook type-A personality. She stated that she wanted to lose weight, tone up, and have the energy to accomplish her intense daily routine. Our sessions would have to be at 5:30 a.m. before she went to work. She had worked with trainers in the past with mixed results, and her exercise routine consisted merely of walking several days a week with friends. She was also a smoker. She had "jogged" for short periods of time in the past but didn't consider herself a runner and had never participated in a race.

We decided that we would work out four times per week: two strength-training sessions and two run sessions. We set a goal of running/walking a 5K race several weeks away. Our initial run sessions consisted of running for a few minutes, walking to recover for a few minutes, and repeating this for thirty minutes or so. We completed the 5K and set our sights on a 10K. She began to lose weight while gaining confidence. Gradually, the running intervals became longer and the walk breaks shorter. We were also running outside in the dead of winter in New England, regardless of weather conditions.

After I paced her to the finish of a 10K and saw her potential to run longer distances, I sprung the idea of a marathon on her moments after crossing the finish line. Not being the type to back down from a challenge, she immediately agreed. We picked a marathon just three months away, established our goal of just finishing the race, and I designed her plan. Because we did not have much time to prepare and she was not capable of completing large amounts of running mileage, I knew that her plan would have to be extremely well balanced and that she would have to be consistent in all the areas. Hence, my Beginner Run 3 Marathon Plan, which includes three runs per week, was born. The basic weekly "cycle" was as follows:

Monday: Full-Body Strength Training

Tuesday: Run/Walk 60 Minutes

Wednesday: Full-Body Strength Training

Thursday: Run/Walk 60 Minutes

Friday: Cross-Train 60 Minutes

Saturday: Long Run (of varying distances)

Sunday: OFF

What was the result? She arrived at the start line injury free. She completed her first marathon with a smile and had an incredible experience. Her initial goal of losing weight was not just achieved but far exceeded. Since then, she has lost even more weight, stopped smoking, completed four more marathons and a triathlon, remained injury free, and made running a part of her life. She plans on running two marathons every year for as long as she is able.

Running three days a week in preparation for a marathon is what I consider to be the very minimum possible. The plan also depends on combining those three runs with at least two days of strength training and one day of quality **cross-training**. But it works, as my client has proven on five occasions and counting!

Cross-training: Engaging in types of exercise other than the primary mode. This can be to rehabilitate an injury, prevent injury, prevent burnout, and maintain and improve fitness.

Most coaches will tell you that you must log a minimum of forty to fifty miles per week to run a marathon. They're wrong. It all comes down to your goals, the quality of your training, your overall program, and your dedication to your plan. If your goal is simply to finish, and you are capable of combining running with strength training and cross-training, then it most certainly can be done. I have extensive real-life proof.

If this is your first marathon, I strongly recommend setting a goal of simply finishing. Setting a time goal as a newbie or first-timer is simply setting yourself up for disappointment and a potentially unpleasant race experience. No matter how you train or how hard you train, trying to achieve a challenging time goal on your first attempt is extremely difficult. So much of the success in endurance racing can be attributed to experience, and as a first-timer you simply do not have the race history that will allow you to choose a fast finishing time. It comes down to pacing, nutrition, hydration, experience, and the weather, just to name a few items. You are much better off choosing the goal of finishing your first race; you can try to improve upon your time in subsequent races.

There are three basic types of goals that can be set when it comes to competition: outcome, performance, and process goals. I utilize all three when it comes to marathon performance and apply them in the following manner.

OUTCOME GOALS

These goals usually involve some type of interpersonal comparison; for marathons, this is most often a finishing time goal. It can also be finishing in a certain place relative to the other participants, such as your overall or age-group place. The difficulty with setting outcome goals is that they can be greatly affected by elements outside your control, such as the race conditions, the course, and your competition for that particular race.

Outcome goals are very difficult to set for people running that distance for the first time. Because they have never experienced that distance before, they tend to set their outcome goal relative to someone else's performance, such as a coworker, a friend, or a family member. "Bill at the office ran the New York City Marathon in four hours and twenty minutes. I know I am in much better shape than he is, so I am going to run my first marathon in just over four hours." Well, maybe, and maybe not. Setting this type of goal is very risky and can result in unpleasant race experiences and misplaced disappointment. Once again, so much about endurance race performance comes down to trial and error, so you cannot expect to run your best race the first time out. Or the second time, or even the third. I have run dozens of marathons, and my last race was my fastest.

Those who have run marathons before often set an outcome goal to better their best race time, to set a **personal record**, or PR. These goals are better than an arbitrary comparison to somebody else's performances, but they are not without potential problems. Your best time may be 4:10, and you may be fitter than you were when you set that time, but a different course and different race-day conditions can slow you down immensely.

Personal record or PR: Your fastest time for a particular distance. This can also be referred to as "personal best," or PB.

Here are some problems associated with outcome goals:

1. *Setting an Unrealistic Outcome Goal:* Let me begin by saying that I am a big believer in pushing the envelope and striving for big goals. I am not someone who believes in always "playing it safe." I even have a hard time with the term "unrealistic." If Roger Bannister, the first person to run the mile in under four minutes, didn't set what was then perceived to be an unrealistic goal, he would not have made it into the history books. There is a big difference, however, in setting "smart" outcome goals and asking too much of yourself too soon. If your best marathon time

is 3:30, attempting to run your next under three hours is a huge leap. Can it be done? Absolutely! Would I bet on it happening? Probably not. Lowering your marathon times is best achieved by a measured progression, and you are better off chipping away at your best time each time. It's also much more enjoyable to better your time by just a little bit each race, if possible. You are constantly improving and slowly teaching your body how to sustain a slightly faster pace each time. Thus, I believe the best type of performance goal to set is simply to improve upon your best time. Not necessarily by five, ten, or twenty minutes, but just to better it. A 4:20 to 4:18 is fine. Five hours to 4:50 is great. What usually happens if you set out to better your time by just one minute is that you may surprise yourself by shaving off more than that. But beating your time is not always possible and can be greatly influenced by the following two factors.

2. *The Course:* All courses are not created equal. Some are much harder than others. A 3:30 on one course may translate to a 3:20 at a different marathon and a 3:45 at yet another, simply due to the layout of the race. Obviously, flatter is generally faster. Chicago is an extremely fast course

because it is pancake flat except for one small hill at the very end. Big Sur is not, because it contains numerous long climbs. I think that the New York City Marathon is much more difficult than most people believe it to be. I personally would therefore not attempt to PR at the NYC Marathon.

You must do your homework and take the layout of the course into account before setting your outcome goal for your next marathon. If your best was on a really flat course, then trying to PR on a really hilly one is probably not such a good idea.

To research the layout of your marathon, you can often go to the race website or the race literature and see the hill profile of your race. The more peaks and valleys there are, the tougher and slower the course will be. If there is one long peak from start to finish, that's bad. If the course profile looks like an EKG of a dead person, that's good.

WARNING: Take all course descriptions of your marathon with a grain of salt. This goes for accounts from race directors, friends, family members, and even strangers. It's one thing to see a definitive visual representation of the course profile; it's quite another to take an individual's personal account of the course. Race directors want to fill their events, so they may take a few liberties with their course descriptions. Official race descriptions of "flat and fast" generally means slightly hilly. "Rolling hills" means be prepared to do some climbing, and "hilly" means look out, you may need Sherpas and supplemental oxygen. Accounts from runners can vary widely: Take no one person's description as gospel.

3. *The Weather:* The weather plays such a huge role in running performance, and much more so than most people realize. High temperatures and humidity can drastically affect you physiologically as well as mentally and can wreak havoc on your race. You may have set an outcome goal based on a marathon you ran in cool, dry conditions, and trying to better that time, even on the very same course, on a much hotter day will be exponentially more difficult. Let's say you ran the Marine Corps Marathon in 4:45 on a 60°F day with low humidity. If the next year you run the race again, but the conditions are 78°F and slightly more humid, running at the same intensity will feel much harder and you will most likely run more slowly, maybe a 5:00 with the very same fitness level. You have to be very smart when it comes to the weather and

your goals. It is crucial that you are able to put your ego aside and be prepared to modify your race goals based on the weather. Many experienced runners seem incapable of doing this, and they suffer as a result. You can train really hard, run your long runs at the appropriate pace, do speed intervals, test yourself at several shorter races, and know that your fitness is right where it needs to be to achieve your performance goal. It is then so difficult to wake up race morning to challenging weather conditions and be forced to completely rethink your race goal. The bottom line is you can't ignore the conditions. The elements will beat you down every time. Thus, your outcome goals can never, ever be set in stone.

Here's a great example of how weather can dramatically affect outcome goals. The Boston Marathon is run in April, so those who train in the Northeast through the cold winter months often find race day to be significantly warmer. Such was the case in 2004. Temperatures climbed to almost 90°F that afternoon, and the course was literally a war zone. Seasoned runners were **blowing up** as early as mile eight, and many were forced to walk even before the halfway point. Local

hospitals admitted a record number of marathoners due to the sweltering conditions. What amazed me was that the majority of these runners knew better than to think they could **hammer** the way they normally did. The fact that most of the runners qualified to run the marathon meant that they had significant race experience. Yet, most refused to readjust their outcome goals and suffered mightily as a result. Why? When I spoke with a veteran runner who was among those who succumbed after running too fast for the elements, he summed it up perfectly. He said he knew it was too hot that day; he knew he should have scrapped his time goal and just run to finish, but as soon as the starting gun went off, two simple words ran through his head: "I'm different." Well, he wasn't so different that day. He was just like all the others who mistakenly believed they could push through the heat and humidity, that they were tougher than everyone else, and that they could stick with their original game plan and outcome goals regardless of weather conditions.

Blowing up: Being forced to slow down considerably during a marathon. While there are multiple causes, blowing up is most often the result of improper pacing, training, nutrition, or hydration, or a combination thereof. A common consequence of blowing up is being forced to finish the race doing the "marathon shuffle," limping along at a snail's pace.

Hammering: Running fast; usually involves passing people.

A very intelligent way to modify your outcome goals because of environmental conditions is to switch from a time-based goal to an overall placement goal. In other words, if you finished in the top 15 percent of the race last year, then your goal might be to finish in the top 14 percent or better on your hot marathon day. This is a smart strategy because everyone will be affected by the conditions, and the average finishing time of all runners will therefore be slower. Running solely against the clock in brutal conditions is courting disaster. Running against the field allows you to accept the elements and adjust for them, yet still have a better outcome than your last race relative to where you finish overall or in your age group.

If you have the discipline to pull back and run against the field in these situations, you will be greatly rewarded. Why? Because most runners are incapable of resetting their goals. They all believe they are "different." They have worked toward a time goal and feel they absolutely, positively must beat it. They have told their family and friends their time goal and do not want to come up short.

I actually love waking up on race morning to find that the conditions are brutally hot and humid. I know that if I just put my ego aside for the first hour or two, I will be passing runners like they are standing still in the later miles. By being patient and adjusting my pace, I am virtually guaranteed to finish much higher in the rankings.

PERFORMANCE GOALS

Performance goals are those that focus on the "strategy" of marathon running. You implement these goals to achieve your outcome goals. Examples of performances goals might be one or more of the following:

1. Walking ten seconds every mile to recover

2. Consuming a gel every thirty minutes

3. Drinking fluids every fifteen minutes

4. Attempting to run **negative splits**

5. Running significantly more slowly during the early miles

6. Keeping your heart rate within a certain zone

7. Not being passed during the final mile

Negative splits: Running the second half of the marathon faster than the first. This is extremely difficult for many to achieve, but, I believe, with proper pacing early on, it is one of the best strategies for the majority of runners to run their fastest times.

Setting intelligent performance goals are crucial to outcome goal attainment. To exponentially increase your chances of hitting your time goal, you must also practice these performance goals throughout your marathon training. Failure to practice performance goals during training is quite often the number one cause of poor performance on race day. You must experiment with these goals over and over to see how your body reacts. This is a long process of trial and error in an attempt to determine cause and effect when it comes to your personal strategy. And it is just that: your personal strategy and no one else's. What works for one person may be a disaster for another.

Once you have assembled your strategy, you must practice it over and over again. As the saying goes, practice doesn't make perfect; perfect practice makes perfect. The goal of training is to approximate your race-day routine as closely as possible. This is essential when it comes to nutrition and hydration. It takes extra thought and effort to plan ahead and carry water, Gatorade, and gels during training, but if you really want to achieve your goals, it is of paramount importance. Shorter races are a great time to practice these strategic elements in a competitive situation. There is an enormous amount of race-day confidence that comes with leaving as few things as possible to chance. It is the little things that count, and in marathon running the little things are practicing your performance goals during training.

PROCESS GOALS

Process goals focus on specific techniques involved in a performance. They almost never need adjusting due to external circumstances, and if you simply implement them, you will by definition always achieve them. Thus, for running, process goals are essentially those techniques that will improve your form and **running economy** including:

1. Running with a soft-foot strike

2. Keeping hands soft and relaxed

3. Keeping shoulders down

4. Keeping arms bent to roughly ninety degrees.

5. Making sure arms swing front to back and not side to side

6. Using gravity on the downhills

7. Utilizing your upper body on the hills

Process goals are often the gaps or weak links in your running form that you need to improve upon. Process goals are also linked to powerful mental tools that I discuss in the chapter on mental training.

Research has shown that the greatest success comes from setting a combination of all three types of goals. The least successful goal-setting strategy is merely to set an outcome goal. This stands to reason, because process goals lead to achieving performance goals, which lead to attaining your outcome goal. Later in the book there will be space for you to write down all three types of goals. Do it. The mere act of writing down your goals will increase the likelihood that you will implement and achieve them.

Running economy: Strictly speaking, it is the oxygen cost of running at a particular speed. Runners who run better, who have better running economy, use less energy running at the same speed as a less economical runner. Therefore, they can run faster for longer periods of time. Running economy has to do with such factors as technique, strength, and flexibility. Improve these and you can improve your running economy.

LOOSE LIPS AND TIMING CHIPS

Once you have decided upon your three types of marathon goals and written them down, I strongly suggest that you keep your outcome goal to yourself. By revealing to others what finishing time you are shooting for, you are potentially adding another unnecessary stressor to your marathon experience. There is really nothing to be gained by telling others how fast you hope to run. If you do run a fast time, even faster than the goal you set, that's great. You and everyone else will be pleasantly surprised. But announcing your time goal to your family and friends can affect both your race-day performance and your enjoyment.

Let's go back to the concept of weather and how it can slow you down considerably given unfavorable conditions. If you have told a bunch of people your time goal, and your marathon conditions turn out to be brutal on race day, you may allow this to cloud your judgment and not adapt accordingly. You know you need to start out slower, hydrate more, and possibly stop for bathroom breaks, but you may refuse to modify your strategy so as not to fail in others' eyes. You essentially give up possession of your outcome goal to other people. This is a true recipe for disaster. You need to control as much of your race as possible and, by announcing your outcome goal, you are essentially bringing others along for the ride who may steer you way off course.

Not only can loose lips influence your race performance, but they can also detract from your race enjoyment. So many things can slow you down, including bad conditions, hitting the wall, a nagging injury, a race-day fall, cramps, and so on. These things happen. When you fall off of your expected pace, you may focus on how you will disappoint everyone who knows your goal rather than concentrate on how to deal effectively with the situation. You spend the rest of the race rehearsing what your story will be about why you fell short of achieving your goal. You focus on negative thoughts instead of positive ones, and this slows you down even more. This can lead to a really negative marathon experience. Endurance races challenge the mind as well as the body; when you are feeling physically fatigued, it is much easier to give up mentally when presented with a reason to do so.

To complicate the matter even further, with the widespread use of **timing chips, timing mats, online athlete trackers**, and even **email and cell phone alerts**, you can literally have an audience watching you race live. You can be halfway around the world while your friends sit home, using their computers to track exactly how your race is unfolding. Well, while you cannot keep others from tracking you during your marathon, you can control their expectations. Your anxiety level will be greatly diminished if you have not revealed your outcome goal to anyone.

It's physiology 101: The less stressed you are, the better you will perform. Stress can increase your heart rate and increase your level of perceived exertion while decreasing your running economy. It can cause you to deviate from your game plan by failing to implement your performance goals and taking your focus off your process goals.

Remember the guy in school who said he didn't study for a test yet aced it, and the guy who told you he was going to get a perfect score and ended up with a 70? Who do you think went into the test feeling more relaxed, with nothing to lose and everything to gain?

When people ask what your time goal is for your marathon, respond that you want to have a "good time", or "just to finish". This goes for first-timers as well as for seasoned veterans. You will enjoy training more, you will enjoy your marathons more, and you will inevitably turn in better times as a result.

Timing chips: Round plastic chips that electronically record your time during a marathon. You generally pick up your chip with your race packet at the marathon expo. You can wear it either tied to your shoelaces or on a strap around your ankle. These chips eliminate the stress about how long it takes you to cross the start line because they begin to record your time when you cross the "timing mat" at the start, not when the gun goes off. As you cross the mat, a computer "reads" your chip, which contains your information. It will record your time when you cross the mats at the start and finish line, and many marathons also place mats at additional points along the course, including the 5K, 10K, half marathon, and 30K markers. You return your chip to a volunteer after crossing the finish line. You can also purchase your own personal chip; it comes with a code that you fill in on your race application, and you can use it at races where chip technology is utilized.

Timing mat: An electronic mat often placed at the start, finish, and various intervals of the marathon or race. The mat receives a signal from a runner's timing chip and records his or her time.

Online athlete tracker: Many marathons have interactive websites where you can track an athlete on race day. Races with this capability allow you to go to the website and input your runner's name; it will then tell you the person's "splits," namely when he or she crossed each timing mat.

Phone and e-mail alerts: In addition to providing online athlete tracking, some races also offer phone and email alerts. You input your phone number and/or your email address, along with the runner (or runners) you wish to follow; a computer will then contact you whenever your athlete crosses a timing mat and provide you with the person's splits.

CHAPTER 3
Keeping an Exercise Journal

One seemingly insignificant habit that yields enormous results is keeping a journal. Writing things down. Some type A personalities are great at this practice, but most of us are not. Studies have corroborated the theory that those who keep records, both dietary and exercise, achieve substantially greater results than those who do not. As runners, we need these journals for our overall success for several reasons:

1. *A Journal Helps "Dial in" Nutrition:* One of the most difficult aspects of sports performance is determining cause and effect: what works for us, what does not, and why. I have found that the vast majority of runners jump to conclusions far too fast, before a true causal relationship can be established. It is therefore crucial to keep a journal detailing as much of your workouts as possible. To be effective runners, we must also be scientists, and every workout is an experiment unto itself. There is, however, a major flaw in each and every one of our experiments. Merriam-Webster defines an experiment as "an operation carried out under controlled conditions." *Controlled* conditions. It is virtually impossible for us to run under truly controlled conditions. Let's say you went out on a training run and consumed vanilla PowerGel for the first time. After experiencing stomach pains during the run, you conclude that vanilla PowerGel caused your gastrointestinal distress. Was it really the PowerGel? Or simply the vanilla-flavored PowerGel? Or was it the consistency of the gel? There are innumerable potential causes of your stomach pains, including:

- What you ate before your run.

- What you didn't eat before your run.

- How close to your run you ate.

- What you drank during your run.

- What you didn't drink during your run.

- Fatigue level.

- Pre-run energy stores.

- The temperature.

- The humidity.

- Your pace.

- When during your run you consumed the PowerGel.

- Whether or not you combined the PowerGel with fluid.

- The difficulty of the terrain.

- Your mental state.

Dial in: Determining what works for you through trial and error.

With so many potential explanations, you must therefore not assign positive or negative qualities to the PowerGel until you have tried it numerous times. This can obviously prove to be problematic, however, because you don't want to continue using something that might be causing your discomfort. That's what makes this whole experimentation process so difficult. There is no perfect way to hydrate or take in food that works for everyone.

So how do you know how many times you should try something before you determine whether it works or not? More than once and less than 100 times. Maybe. It all depends on how well you design your "experiments," how much data you compile, and how well you can interpret the results. Unfortunately, there is no precise number because the other variables change with each run. This is why keeping written records is such a key part of your "scientific process." By chronicling the major elements of each run, you will slowly begin to see patterns emerge. The operative word here is slowly.

Back to the PowerGel: Let's say you tried it on five runs and each time you experienced similar stomach distress. Then you ran three times without the gel and felt better. You still ought not to assign blame to the gel, but it is a good start. You may try taking in pieces of an energy bar during subsequent runs and experience the exact same distress. You may experiment with different flavors, foods, and forms of food (liquid, semisolid, and solid) and vary the point in your runs when you take them in. The more consistent you are with your journal, the more data you compile, and the more you will gradually be able to dial in your own individualized nutritional strategy.

I realize that many people may complain that keeping a journal is too much work. Well, the few minutes it may take to scribble down notes after each run will produce massive dividends in the long term. Write down what you eat before a run, how much, and when. Write down what you drink during a run, how much, and when. Do the same for any semisolid and solid foods, and you will be well on your way to figuring out your optimal nutritional strategy.

Note: Realize that this experimentation is a never-ending process. I have run hundreds of races and I am still tweaking my nutritional strategy. Once you have a firm foundation from which to work, however, you will find yourself focused more on refining and fine-tuning. Just be sure not to change what works for you in an attempt to improve performance even more.

You must also realize that race day will present a whole host of new elements that you could not prepare for in your training. In other words, on race day you will experience the following, which were not part of your training:

- Adrenaline
- Spectators
- Running with thousands of runners
- Fear
- Anxiety
- Outcome goals
- The course (if you have not run it before)
- Current fitness status

Any one of these factors can affect your race performance enormously; combine two or more and you are in for a completely different "experiment" altogether. This is why it is crucial to practice, practice, practice with all the strategies you intend to use during your marathon. Although you cannot truly duplicate the race-day elements listed above, you need to feel as comfortable as possible with your plan, and your journal will be instrumental for this. These race-day factors can confuse your tested strategy, and you may assign blame to something that was not the actual cause. People have told me how they ate something during their marathon and by mile twenty they felt horrible. Was it really what they ingested or could it have been their marathon pacing, their pre-race energy stores, or the fact that they may not have consumed enough of that specific food? This is why so much of marathon running comes down to marathon experience. Race-day conditions are so different from those of training that it takes running many marathons before you can dial in what works for you on race day as well. You should not expect to have your best race the first time out. You should not expect your race to unfold exactly as you planned. You should, however, use your journal to record detailed notes on all aspects of your marathon experience for extensive review after your race and for comparison to future races.

Note: So much about endurance racing success lies in proper "fueling." This includes post-workout, and before, duirng, and after the race itself. Our bodies generally do not seem to want to consume foods when we are moving, especially at higher rates of speed; however, fuel intake is essential for achieving our goals. From my personal experience and from coaching clients, I find that most people need to feel some level of race-day discomfort as a result of proper nutrition and hydration. It is my philosophy that it is much better to feel a little queasy during your marathon than to become dehydrated or energy-depleted. You can run through queasiness and often it will pass; dehydration and **bonking** will not. Don't rush to judgment when experimenting with your fuel intake.

Bonk: The same as hitting the wall; being forced to slow way down during an endurance event. It is usually accompanied by major fatigue and lightheadedness. It is primarily due to fuel (glycogen) depletion but can be caused by a combination of factors, including poor training, dehydration, heat, and improper pacing.

2. *A Journal Helps Prevent Injuries:* Once again, running does not cause injuries; it illuminates our weak links and shows us what we need to work on. If you experience pain from running yet continue to follow the same program, you will most likely become injured. Although I am injury free, that does not mean that some type of pain does not present itself during my training. The moment I feel a twinge or soreness, I immediately set about trying to diagnose the cause and fix it before it becomes a real problem. Keeping a running journal is essential in this diagnostic process. When you record your workouts, along with all relevant information, you can begin to narrow down the possible causes. So many running injuries come from doing too

much too soon or from increasing your mileage too quickly. Your journal will allow you to look back at your training to see where the possible cause may lie.

Let's say you began to experience knee pain while going up and down stairs. You look back at your journal and see that you ran twenty miles one week, twenty-two miles the next, twenty-four miles the third week, and thirty-six miles on the fourth. The jump of twelve miles from week three to week four is a big one and could possibly have brought about the knee soreness. You would therefore pull back the following week to allow your body to rest and recover.

Now let's say you experienced the same type of knee pain and looked back at your journal only to find that you did not increase your mileage substantially from one week to the next. So you examine your notes further. You notice that you bought a new brand and style of training shoe the week before. If you try running on your old pair for a week and the pain subsides, the new shoes may be to blame.

Finally, maybe you experience the same type of knee pain and examine your notes. No real mileage issues and no changes of footwear. You do see, however, that on your cross-training days you switched from swimming to riding a stationary bike. Maybe an incorrect seat position or another bike-related issue is the cause of the problem. You go back to swimming on your cross-training days and the pain gradually disappears; potential injury avoided.

A journal is so important in helping to diagnose and prevent injuries. It is next to impossible to remember exactly how many miles we log each week over the course of many months, what numerous variations we add to our training, such as speed and hill work, and subtle changes like new running shoes. Quite often, small changes can disrupt the balance of your body in a big way, and by recording all these elements, you can take control of your training in a major way.

3. *A Journal Can Determine Optimal Training Volume:* Running is a never-ending "experiment of one" and therefore highly individualistic. After running different amounts of miles each week, you begin to realize what works for you. If you are a veteran of several marathons, this information is invaluable in determining what works for you and what does not. Let's say

that you have run three marathons: a 4:15, a 3:55, and a 4:30, in that order. When you study your notes, you see that you ran on average fifty miles per week for your 4:15 finish, forty per week for your time of 3:55, and you pushed yourself and jumped up to sixty-plus miles per week for your marathon time of 4:30. Once again, marathon performance is incredibly multifactorial and you cannot ascribe definitive cause and effect to any single element. It may have been significantly hotter on the day you ran your 4:30 than on the prior two marathons. You can, however, examine this type of data and hypothesize that you may have overtrained for that slower finish. More is not necessarily better, especially when it comes to endurance training. You may decide to return to running around forty miles per week for your next marathon. If your performance is significantly better, you may then have an idea of the amount of **training volume** that serves you best.

Training volume: The amount of miles you run. Usually computed by week, it is the total number of miles you run from Monday through Sunday. The amount of training volume you need is based on numerous factors, including your marathon goals, current fitness status, and personal physiological and biomechanical makeup.

4. *A Journal Builds Confidence:* Training for a marathon takes months, and we often have short memories when it comes to exactly what we did during our training. Your running journal will be very important for your confidence at two distinct times in your marathon training: during the taper phase and the night before your race.

During the taper phase, you will dramatically scale back your training for several weeks leading up to marathon day. This can be extremely difficult for many runners to do, both physically and mentally. They have invested so much time in their training and they believe that if they decrease their training volume, they will lose fitness and their performance will suffer. In fact, the exact opposite is true, but you often cannot reason with a runner experiencing the effects of taper. I believe that a failure to adequately scale back running miles during the last few weeks of training is a top reason that runners do not achieve their true potential. This is where the running journal can help. You will spend time during your taper phase rereading your journal, as if it were a novel. You will be amazed at the number of workouts you forgot about; that miserable twenty-miler in the pouring rain, all those speedwork sessions, those strength-training workouts, that half marathon you ran and posted your fastest time ever, and so on. By revisiting your months of training and recalling the totality of your efforts, you will be less likely to overdo it during the final weeks. A true taper is vital to marathon success yet so very difficult a concept for most to implement effectively. The running journal can be the device by which you avoid sabotaging all your hard efforts, allowing you to rest, recover, and arrive at the start line perfectly refreshed.

Your journal will also boost your confidence immeasurably the night before your race. After you have laid out your race outfit, attached your chip to your shoe, assembled all your gear, and packed your bag, you will sit down with your running diary one last time. Flipping through the pages, you will absorb all the hard work you have accomplished in the past several months. You will see in black and white all the long runs you completed, all the crunches you counted, and all the

minutes you spent stretching. You will realize that you have controlled all that you can and that you are absolutely ready for the next day's race. The weather won't matter because you have trained in all kinds of elements. You are comfortable in your hydration and nutritional strategy because it has been tested over and over again. You will go to bed confident that you have prepared as best you could, looking forward to the next day's payoff and the chance to reap the rewards of your training.

Marathon racing is challenging by definition. Things will inevitably go wrong, and you will most likely experience some degree of discomfort on race day. This is all part of the allure and the thrill of running a marathon. If it were easy, finishing wouldn't be half as rewarding. By spending just a few minutes after each workout keeping an exercise journal, you will exponentially increase your race performance as well as your race enjoyment for many years to come.

Note: In 2005, the average age of marathon runners was 36.1 for women and 40.5 for men.

GEAR

One of the things I love about running is its simplicity. All you need is a pair of sneakers and you are good to go. No matter where you are in the world, you can lace up your shoes and go out for a run. Some of the most amazing sightseeing I have done has been on exploratory runs in such places as Malaysia, South Korea, Germany, New Zealand, and Australia.

Although a pair (or two) of good running sneakers is the main requirement for runners, needs change as distances get longer. The type of clothing we wear, along with additional gear, can make us go faster and longer while providing greater comfort.

This section on gear appears early for a reason. One of the keys to endurance racing is to make your practice as similar to race day as possible. In other words, on race day you want everything you are wearing to have been tested beforehand, ideally during numerous workouts. Disaster can strike during your race due to a seemingly insignificant, minute change to your race wear. You do not want to leave anything to chance. And just because something worked during shorter training runs does not mean that it will work on runs of fifteen miles or more. As we run longer, there is a strange phenomenon that happens to our bodies and to our clothing and gear

as well, and you do not want to experience it for the first time on race day. These are two extremely important concepts of marathon running. First: You must road test all gear on runs of fifteen miles or more before anything can be deemed race-worthy. And second, what I consider to be the absolute first commandment of marathon running: Thou shall not try anything on race day that thee have not done in practice. Anything.

Before I cover running gear, let me first share just one example of how breaking the first commandment can affect your marathon performance. It happened to me during the tenth anniversary of my first Boston Marathon race.

During the 2002 Boston Marathon I changed my race outfit the night before the race. I decided to wear a pair of shorts that I had never run long in together with a pair of spandex shorts underneath. I had, in fact, run in both items before but never for more than six miles or so. Well, all was fine for the first half marathon. It was a beautiful Monday in Massachusetts, perhaps a little warm for a marathon, but I enjoy the heat. I am also a heavy sweater, so I was dripping as the race progressed. My shorts were made of a thicker fabric than the shorts I normally raced in, and the elastic waistband was a little bit on the loose side. You may see where this is going. As the race went on, I sweated more and more and my shorts were working overtime soaking it all up. As I sprinted past the cheering students of my alma mater at Boston College, unbeknownst to me, the law of gravity was waging a heavy battle with the coefficient of **friction** on the lower half of my body. I made my way down into Cleveland Circle and, right when I was passing Mary Ann's, a popular Boston College dive bar, before a full audience lining the front of the establishment, the law of gravity won. My shorts plummeted down to my ankles and I stumbled to keep from falling. The onlookers were treated to quite a show as I attempted to pull my drenched shorts back up without breaking stride. When I had my shorts back around my waist, I realized that the elastic waistband was no longer elastic and, if I let go of them, they would drop once again. Not willing to shed the sweat-soaked shorts and finish down Beacon Street wearing nothing but a thin layer of spandex, I spent the final miles of the marathon running while holding up my shorts with both hands—not a particularly good look, nor a technique for improving running economy and speed.

Friction: (1) The rubbing of one body against another; (2) The force that resists relative motion between two bodies in contact. As marathon runners, we want to eliminate as much of this "resistance" as possible. Friction is your worst enemy.

The following is a discussion of the gear associated with marathon running. You won't need all of it; you will experiment and determine what works best for you. Many gear choices are determined by personal goals, nutritional and hydration needs, comfort, and plain old personal preference.

Just as you will experiment with your nutrition during training, you will also experiment with your clothing and gear. The closer you get to race day, however, the less you will experiment. By then, you should have tried everything on numerous occasions during your training to ensure that it will work for you during your marathon. The sooner you dial in your marathon clothing and gear, the better. Once again, this serves to guard against unforeseen problems, and it also leads to increased confidence. The more miles you can log using the exact strategies that you will engage in during your marathon, the more comfortable and self-assured you will be at the starting line.

Running Shoes

Common sense tells you that one of the most important pieces of running equipment is your running shoes. The difficultly lies in the fact that that there is no single "best" shoe. I am constantly asked what the best running shoe is, and my short answer is always the same: whichever works best for you. Choosing the right running shoe is based on numerous criteria, including your goals, weekly running mileage, and individual **biomechanics**.

Biomechanics: The mechanics of biological and especially muscular activity, as in locomotion and exercise.

Essentially, this means that because we are all built differently, we all have different needs when it comes to footwear. This is one area where the maxim "What works for one person will not necessarily work for another" is especially true. Just because your friend says he absolutely, positively loves Brand X and you have to get them doesn't mean that it is the correct footwear for you. A few criteria involved in selecting the correct running shoe include the following:

- Your weekly running mileage
- Your arch type: high, normal, or flat
- Your weight
- Your foot width
- The rolling motion of your foot: pronator, supinator, or neutral
- Whether you are using them for training or racing
- Your goal race distance
- Your training and race terrain

Choosing the correct running shoe should be left to the experts. This means that you should purchase your shoes from a store that specializes in running shoes and is staffed by runners. I believe it is imperative that you buy your shoes in a store whose primary product is running shoes. Not tents, guns, surfboards, or basketball nets. Running shoes.

Note: Some specialty running stores now have treadmills, so a salesperson can examine your "gait," or how you run, to help determine the best running shoe for you.

A qualified running-store employee should ask you numerous questions, touching on the areas listed above. He or she should also inquire as to what shoes, if any, you currently run in. If you currently own running shoes, wear or bring them along so the salesperson can examine the soles to see the wear pattern. The salesperson should measure your feet regardless of the size shoe you wear. The more questions the salesperson asks, the better. Although you should trust your running-store salesperson to be knowledgeable and to choose the appropriate shoe for you, the following are some basics of the science of running shoes.

Running-shoe manufacturers have three basic categories of shoes: cushioning, stability, and motion control. There can be a great deal of variation within these categories, but this is generally where you begin your shoe selection. Here are brief definitions of the three categories:

1. Cushioning shoes have little lateral support, or support from side to side. They are generally for people who have "neutral feet" and a high arch. Runners who "supinate" will often wear cushioning shoes.

2. Stability shoes offer a balance between cushioning and motion control. Runners with normal arches who land on the outside of their feet will generally choose stability shoes.

3. Motion control shoes are for runners who need support. Just as their name implies, these shoes control feet that "pronate" excessively upon foot strike.

Running Times magazine estimates that 80 percent of runners are categorized as overpronators. What exactly is "pronation"

and "supination" and how do you know whether you do one or the other? And if you pronate or supinate, how do you know whether you do so excessively? Once again, you should leave these determinations to your running-store professional, but the following briefly explains the "rolling" mechanisms of our feet.

Our feet roll to the inside and to the outside when we run; this is a necessary component of proper locomotion. Only when we do too much of one or the other do problems occur. Pronation happens when our foot rolls inward; supination is when it rolls outward. The reason a good running-shoe salesperson will examine your current shoes is that the wear on the soles is evidence of your individual running pattern. Most of the wear should begin on the outside of your heels. If the wear on the forefoot is predominantly on the medial, or inside, of your shoe, you may be an overpronator. If the lateral, or outside, of your shoe has the greatest amount of wear, underpronation may be occurring. "Neutral" feet create equal wear across the forefoot.

You can determine which type you have by performing the simple "wet test." Wet your feet and then stand on a flat, dry paper bag. Step off and the imprints will show you your individual arch type.

Runners with normal arches are generally neutral pronators. Those with low arches are usually associated with overpronation, and people with high arches are prone to supination and underpronation.

I prefer to leave my footwear choices to the professionals in the running stores. I train in the same shoes that I race in, and I have found great success with this strategy.

Years ago, I decided that I wanted to change my running shoes. I walked into a running store in New York City and informed the salesperson of this fact. He asked me what shoes I currently ran in and then asked what was wrong with them. I replied that nothing was wrong with them, that I merely wanted a change. He suggested that if my shoes weren't giving me any problems, I should buy a new pair of the exact same shoe. Looking back, I realize how smart and honest that salesperson was. He very easily could have offered me the most expensive shoe on the market and regaled me with all of its impressive attributes. Instead, he illustrated one of the cardinal rules of marathon running: If it works, stick with it.

Remember my analogy of how we as runners are akin to scientists, endlessly performing experiments in an attempt to uncover our personal strategies and formulas? If you are fortunate enough to find something that really works for you, you should not change it for the mere sake of doing so.

When it comes to your gear, you must not choose something simply because it "looks good." The shorts I wore at the 2002 Boston Marathon looked great (for a time) but performed horribly. Shoe manufacturers often change the color of their shoes from year to year. You should not change shoes simply because they used to be blue and now they are green and you love green. If the shoe fits, wear it, and if it works for you, keep it, regardless of how ugly it may be.

Note: Marathon gear choices are to be made based on function, not fashion.

Finally, do not seek out the cheapest shoe to save money. Your shoes are the most important component of your marathon gear: Take care of your feet and your feet will take care of you. You are asking your feet to perform under stressful conditions, and you need to prepare them accordingly. Likewise, do not try to save money by running in old, worn-out shoes as you postpone purchasing new ones. The rule of thumb is that you should replace your running shoes every 300 to 500 miles (another great reason to keep a running journal), and I would err on the conservative side and replace them every 350 miles or so. Quite often you will reach this 350-mile mark even before your shoes look too worn. My experience has shown that if your running shoes look old, you've been running in them too long. A strategy used by many runners is to buy two pairs at a time and rotate them.

CLOTHING

There have been great advances in clothing since I ran my first marathon in 1992 wearing an old cotton Boston College T-shirt. What amazes me is how many people continue to exercise and run in clothing that negatively affects their performance and detracts from their comfort. The longer you run, the more poor clothing choices can affect you.

The following is a list of attributes that you should look for in your running clothing, including socks, shorts, shirts, and hats:

1. Lightweight
2. Breathable
3. Antifriction
4. Antimicrobial
5. Moisture-wicking
6. Fast-drying

Coolmax is a popular fabric that is great for performance wear. Coolmax fabrics are designed to keep you feeling cool and dry by "wicking" moisture away from your body and increasing the garment's drying rate.

This is something that cotton does not do and something that is essential for runners, especially in hot and humid conditions.

Other name-brand technical fabrics include Supplex, Micromattique, Polartec, and Power Dry. And polyester, that '70s fashion faux pas, is now your friend as a marathon runner. Much of the quality running performance clothing is either 100 percent polyester or polyester blended with such fabrics as spandex. You can purchase tank tops, short-sleeve or long-sleeve shirts, and even jackets made from these performance materials. Don't underestimate the importance of wearing the correct materials when you run, especially during a marathon.

Note: As of June 26, 2006, the oldest man to complete a marathon is Dimitrion Yordandis, ninety-eight, and the oldest woman is ninety-one-year-old Jenny Wood-Allen.

RUNNING SHORTS

Marathoners run in a wide variety of running shorts. The split-short, with its slit up the sides and short length, was very popular in the early days of marathoning. Although some runners still prefer this style, others have found it to be too revealing, and the loose fabric can lead to chafing. Once again, you should choose shorts that are lightweight and breathable and made with a wicking fabric. Remember that you need to base your decision on what feels good, not necessarily what looks good. You don't want shorts to be too long or too baggy because these tend to bunch up and lead to chafing, especially as you sweat. You definitely want to experiment with different running shorts to determine what works best for you. I have found through much trial and error that I run best in spandex shorts, either alone or underneath very basic lightweight running shorts. The tight spandex helps eliminate potential chafing, and I have found great success with this strategy. If I do decide to run "spandex only," depending on the conditions, my well-positioned race number on my race belt affords me the "frontal cover" I need.

Some shorts come with liners inside; others do not. This is a personal choice on your part. Many have tiny inside pockets that are perfect for carrying small items on your runs; the pockets are especially helpful on longer runs, when you need money to buy food and drinks, or if you bonk and need to pay for transportation home. There are shorts that have numerous pockets on the outside for storing your keys, gels, bars, and other items during your training runs and your marathon. One brand that specializes

in these types of multi-pocketed apparel is RaceReady. I have not tried these garments and prefer to carry my stuff either on a belt or in a flask in my hand, be careful not to overload your shorts too much. Inevitably, runners who do will fail to practice running long distances with their shorts heavily loaded only to encounter major problems during the marathon.

If you like to run early in the morning or later at night, select shorts with reflective properties for safety purposes.

SOCKS

Sock choice may seem insignificant, but it certainly is not. I seem to be able to run without any socks (though I don't recommend this, if just for shoe odor sake) or with a wide variety of sock types. Other runners swear by a certain sock brand and, if it works for them, that's what they will use. Generally speaking, you want to find a sock that is thin and breathable and made from a technical fabric. Do not run in thick, heavy cotton socks. Some may believe that thick socks provide padding and comfort over the long haul, but that's precisely what your shoes should deliver. Thick socks can overheat your feet and result in blister formation. Find a lightweight pair, wear them while being fitted for your running shoes, and then purchase several pairs and rotate them. Friction is one of your worst enemies as a marathoner, so you want to do whatever possible to minimize the points of friction all over your body—especially in your feet. You can accomplish this by wearing clothing that fits correctly, choosing performance fabrics, and buying anti-chafing products. One small blister can ruin your race, and performance-wear socks will help reduce the chance of blisters forming.

SHIRTS AND TOPS

There is an enormous variety of running shirts to choose from for both men and women. Running stores are packed with a seemingly infinite array of colors and styles: tank tops, sleeveless, compression wear, and much more. You should select shirts with the same characteristics as your performance socks: lightweight, breathable, antimicrobial, moisture-wicking, and fast-drying. And please, no cotton! Cotton keeps the moisture close to your skin; performance fabrics wick it away to keep you cooler and drier. This means that wearing the official cotton marathon shirt you received in your race bag is a no-no during the race. That is, unless you're running a marathon like Big Sur. When my father and I ran this absolutely breathtaking marathon in 2004, each runner was provided with a top-quality performance-wear race shirt.

Note: Among the newest types of clothing for athletes and runners is compression clothing. Made popular by UnderArmour, these garments are skintight and made from performance materials. While many may not feel comfortable wearing this alone, compression clothing can be great as an underlayer when you wear more than one layer, especially in colder conditions.

2005 Marathon Statistics

Age Group	Avg. Time
M0–19	5:04:39
M20–24	4:22:21
M25–29	4:24:42
M30–34	4:25:28
M35–39	4:22:45
M40–44	4:21:46
M45–49	4:26:23
M50–54	4:37:25
M55–59	4:49:04
M60+	5:13:32
F0–19	5:46:58
F20–24	4:52:38
F25–29	4:54:45
F30–34	4:58:18
F35–39	4:55:37
F40–44	4:59:01
F45–49	5:11:46
F50–54	5:31:03
F55–59	5:48:39
F60+	6:08:12

Source: www.marathonguide.com

Note: In 2006, I introduced my new TeamHolland Apparel line of fitness wear. All garments are created using the best materials and latest technology. The shorts, shirts, and jackets are designed for maximum comfort without being too anything—too bright, too tight, too hot, too short, or too outdated. To see the line, visit www.teamholland.com and click on Apparel.

HEADWEAR

Not long ago, a friend showed me some notes her marathon coach provided to his training clients. One of the statements he made was that clients were not to wear any type of hat during the marathon because it would trap body heat and make them hotter as a result. Not necessarily true. Yes, during a hot marathon, you would not want to wear a winter wool cap on your head, but a performance hat or visor can boost your performance. Wicking hats made form Coolmax or Coolmax-type materials are washable, breathable, and moisture wicking, and they keep the sun off your head and the sweat out of your eyes. You can wet them down with water or even put ice cubes in them during extremely hot races. Similarly, visors will help keep the sun off your face and out of your eyes. The mere act of squinting for

twenty-six miles can create tension in the face and waste valuable energy.

I always say that if you want to know what to do when it come to racing strategy, just look to the best and imitate them. So, when it comes to what to wear during endurance races, I look to the elites, especially the top finishers at the Hawaii Ironman Triathlon. This race is run in the extremes of heat and humidity. The vast majority of professionals wear something on their heads, whether it is a hat, visor, or bandanna-type head covering. Having the sun beat down on your head and face while exerting yourself for three to six hours can really take a toll on you. Wearing a hat while running in challenging conditions can help improve your marathon performance.

A Run to the Sun
One of my most special race experiences to date was my first ultramarathon, the 36-mile *Run to the Sun* on the island of Maui. Billed as the only point-to-point marathon where you can see the finish from the start, the race began at sea level and finished at the 10,023-foot summit of the volcano Mount Haleakala. The challenging course is said to be the steepest paved road on Earth, and, because it is sponsored in part by H.U.R.T., the Hawaii Ultra Running Team, you just know it's not going to be an easy day.

The experience was utterly spectacular. The race began at the Maui shopping center at 4:30 a.m. in the pitch dark. By the light of the moon, you could just barely make out the silhouette of Mount Haleakala off in the distance. There was a small group attempting this unique ultramarathon, and as the starting gun rang out and we set off toward the base of the volcano, it was so dark that I often found myself struggling just to make out the road in front of me. The voices of unseen runners drifted through the warm Hawaiian air and disappeared into the silence. On several occasions the black sky was illuminated by the most brilliant shooting stars that I have ever seen. After running roughly ten kilometers, the soft morning light eased through the darkness and we began our slow ascent up the volcano. The road snaked up Mount Haleakala in a never-ending series of switchbacks leading toward a seemingly unreachable summit. The volcano is probably best known for the group bike rides that take place at sunrise from the summit down to the bottom; these riders passed me every so often, and I ran by several groups stopped on the roadside who watched me with silent wonder as I slowly trudged by.

As I rounded what seemed like the 200th switchback, I saw what appeared to be fog covering the road ahead. Approaching this thick "fog," I passed a road sign that read, "Please turn on your headlights in the clouds."

"Clouds?"

I believe it was at that moment that I felt as if I had just sucked in several dozen helium balloons.

I was in a respectable fifth place at this point, but not for much longer. I had read all about altitude and its effects on the human body during exercise, but this was my first experience with it. At roughly 8,000 feet I approached a much needed aid station staffed by two smiling twenty-somethings. I'm not sure whether they were smiling because they were having a good time or whether it was an attempt to hold back uncontrollable laughter at how I looked: I was absolutely dripping with sweat, staggering up the side of the road, shirtless, sunburned, and with the ever-present smile on my face. As I slowed to a crawl, they asked how I felt, and I replied, "Great! What a day!" They then asked if I needed anything and I told them I was dying for a cup of ice. They quickly produced one and handed it to me. I thanked them and set off "running" again. I was going to use the ice as I had in dozens of prior races in the extreme heat: I would dump it into my hat and put the hat back on my head. Melting ice is extremely effective in cooling down the body, and the scorching Hawaiian sun seemed to be getting closer and closer.

For this race, I had slightly changed my race attire during training. As the two aid station volunteers looked on, I removed my visor, dumped the ice through it onto the pavement, put the visor back on and kept running, all without missing a step. I'm pretty sure I heard them radio to the next aid station and tell them to check on me when I arrived, but I quite possibly may have hallucinated that.

The altitude absolutely crushed me the last few miles. My routine became: run hard for a few steps, almost pass out, slow down, feel my heart move into my throat, repeat. Several runners passed me as I struggled toward the summit, which crushed me even further because one of my performance goals is to try never to be passed in the final miles of a race. As I crept toward the finish line, the surroundings turned into what looked like the surface of the moon: barren, black rock for as far as the eye could see. Another bad sign.

I finally crossed the finish line in ninth place and received a truly special handmade finisher's medal. The "Run to the Sun" was among the toughest and most magical races I have ever competed in. A week later, I ran the Boston Marathon, and Heartbreak Hill seemed like a mere speed bump.

SUNGLASSES

Along with your hat or visor, wearing sunglasses can be yet another way to decrease the tension in your face caused by the glare on sunny marathon days. Our goal as marathoners is to make running as easy as possible, and every little bit of help counts. You can place glasses on the brim of your hat or visor when you don't need them and pull them down when the conditions warrant.

FUEL BELTS

Marathon running requires intelligent nutrition and hydration, both during training and on race day. This can be difficult to do, especially in training. During your marathon, you can get water and electrolyte drinks from the numerous aid stations positioned throughout the course, but you may also want to supplement this with your own supplies. There are obviously no aid stations during your longer practice runs, so you will need to carry food, drinks, and various other items with you. What's the best way to do this? Once again, much of what you decide to do will be based on your personal preference. There are a wide variety of products to choose from as well as ways to transport needed energy sources and fluids. The bottom line is that you must at the very least take in fluids during your longer runs.

Note: It seems that the faster you run, the less fluid and energy requirements you need, if for no other reason than you are running for a shorter period of time. However, this does not mean that you do not need extra fuel just because you are a faster runner. Those running five- and six-hour marathons may require more fuel both in training and on race day, but just because the elites don't carry additional energy doesn't mean you don't need to.

Fuel Belt, from the company that pioneered the multi-bottle hydration belt, is one of the most popular beverage and nutritional carrying systems. Theses belts are ideal for storing fluids and gels in ergonomically designed bottles. They also have Velcro-closure pockets that are ideal for carrying additional small items such as electrolyte tablets, aspirin, small portions of food, money, and keys. Many runners use these belts both in training and during the race. Remember that you want to make your training resemble your marathon as much as possible, so whatever you do during your long training runs you should also do during your marathon.

Even though there are aid stations on the marathon course, there are several reasons to wear something like a Fuel Belt:

1. *You May Want Your Own Type of Fluid:* Races contract with beverage sponsors that provide the fluids for the aid stations. You may not like that particular brand or that particular flavor and wish to consume your own tried and tested fluids.

2. *Energy Gels Are Rarely Provided:* Many runners will want to consume a certain number of energy gels during their marathon. Races rarely provide these gels, and if they do, they usually hand them out at the later miles of the race, when it may be too late. You can either fill these bottles with gels premixed with fluid or fill up one or more entirely with gel.

3. *It Is Always Better to Be "Self-Contained":* In other words, you should never expect that fluids and food will be available to you on race day. Aid stations have been known to run out of supplies such as water, electrolyte drinks, and food. In the more crowded races you can often become swept up in the masses and miss an aid station due to congestion. You may also want fuel in between stations. Thus, it is always better to have what you need on you than to depend on it being provided at just the right moment.

These belts come in a variety of styles with different numbers of bottles, bottle shapes, and add-ons. There are "hydration packs," where you carry the water on your back and sip it through an attached straw. There are also belts that carry one or more full-size water bottles. Although these designs are made for as much comfort as possible, I find them to be a little more cumbersome. Some marathon runners who use the run/walk strategy prefer to use the full-size water bottles so they can bring more fluids with them.

I will repeat this point concerning training and racing throughout the book because it is so important: If you plan on using a Fuel Belt or any other fuel-carrying device during your marathon, be sure to train with it during your long runs and then stick with that exact one on race day. As well constructed as this equipment is, it can still rub and chafe you. You want to be sure you have achieved the perfect fit and have road tested the product many times before taking it twenty-six miles.

For example, I observed a runner at a recent marathon who had pinned her gels to her shorts. She was wearing a sports bra with her midsection exposed and you could see that she was bleeding in several places on her back, spots where the gels were bouncing and rubbing against her skin. It was mile eighteen, and several hours of constant chafing had taken its toll. Remember that you want to minimize rubbing on all parts of your body; everything should be secured tightly without being uncomfortable.

2005 Marathon Statistics

	Percent	Avg. Age	Avg. Time
Men	60.0%	40.5	4:32:08
Women	40.0%	36.1	5:06:08
All Runners	100.0%	38.7	4:45:00

Source: www.marathonguide.com

RACE NUMBER BELTS

The most common way to affix your marathon race number to your body is with four small safety pins that you receive in your registration bag. You generally place a pin in each corner of your race number and attach it to the front of your shirt. Do not attach it to your back; this is against the rules and you will miss out on your pictures if your number is not visible from the front (race photographers snap pictures at various points during the marathon and identify you by the race number on your front). I recommend using a race belt instead of the safety-pin method. These belts are just that: belts you wear around your waist and attach your marathon number to, usually with two snaps. One reason to use a race belt is that quite often you may change during a marathon, adding or removing clothing layers. If you attach your race number to your shirt and then decide you want to shed that layer, you must also take off and reaffix the number, which can be a time-consuming nuisance.

Note: In 2005, there were a total of 314 marathons held in the U.S.

WATCHES

There has been a virtual explosion in running-watch technology in the past decade. No longer do watches simply keep time; you now can buy entire watch "systems" that display distance traveled, heart rate, speed, calories burned, and much more, and you can upload this information to your computer for analysis or future reference, or to e-mail to your coach. Some watches use a calibration system to compute your distance and speed; others use the Global Positioning System (GPS) to gather this data. These watches are synchronized with satellites to track your route and measure your speed and distance. There are several different systems on the market today. Polar, one of the leaders in sport-watch and heart-rate technology, offers one with a foot pod that provides you with accurate heart rate, running pace, and distance information without having to rely on satellites.

Garmin, a leader in GPS technology, offers several watch options, including the Forerunner 301. The 301 continuously monitors your heart rate, speed, distance, pace, and calories burned, along with a whole host of additional features. Because it relies on satellites, there is no foot pod or calibration required.

Timex also offers several styles of running-watch systems that utilize GPS technology. I personally use the Timex Bodylink System and love it. It is so easy to use and also extremely accurate. So which watch should you buy? That choice is completely up to you, and, depending on your marathon goals, you might not even need a watch at all! Everything depends on your goals and your personality type. Obviously, the more data you have, the better able you are to monitor your training and track your progress. One great feature of watches that measure distance is that you can just go out and run wherever you feel like; you don't have to measure the route before or after, and you can pick your route as you go. This is especially helpful when you travel or if you like to run on trails. The ability to upload your training data to your computer is also a valuable feature because it helps to compile an "electronic running journal" for future reference.

Just remember that no matter how good your gear is, nothing can take the place of consistent training. I have seen far too many runners get bogged down in heart rate training and meticulously tracking their data rather than focusing on what really counts—

getting in the miles. I remain a big fan of the most basic and most popular watches, such as the Timex Ironman, with a simple stopwatch to record runs. For those runners who wish to train by heart rate, simpler is often better. The dizzying array of features offered by the more expensive heart-rate watches rarely get used, and the real-time heart rate display is the sole function most runners need. The Polar FS1 is a simple and easy-to-use entry-level monitor.

One of the benefits of purchasing any of these watches and systems is that it tends to lead to increased adherence to your running program. Using these products can add a new dimension to your training and make your workouts more fun. The distance systems will allow you to explore new running routes while still providing an accurate record of the miles you travel.

Note: In 2003, comedian and actor Will Ferrell ran the Boston Marathon in 3:56:12.

MUSIC

I am a huge fan of listening to music while I run, especially on those long solitary Sunday endurance workouts. I tend to run alone the majority of the time and my music is a welcome companion. I mix it up as well; some runs I want to be alone with my thoughts, while other days I wish to be distracted and entertained. Although I attempted to listen to music during my first marathon, I now prefer to utilize it solely during training. There is an interesting concept that has been studied in runners that deals with "association" and "dissociation." Research has shown that new runners tend to want to "disassociate" during their runs, essentially having their minds taken away from the task at hand. They want to think about anything other than the fact that they are running, and music is a great tool for accomplishing this. As runners become more experienced and wish to run faster, however, there is a switch toward a need and desire to "associate" and focus on the process of running. These runners need to monitor their breathing, pace, form, and so forth to achieve their goals.

When I brought along music during that first marathon, it was a cassette-playing Walkman that was the size of a brick and almost as heavy. Technology has come a long way since 1992, cassettes have been replaced by digital music players, and the options for running with music are amazing. The players are as lightweight and small as can be, with the capacity to hold an incredible amount of music. Apple's iPod is one of the most popular means of exercising with tunes, and these devices get smaller yet more powerful every year. By the time this book is published, iPods will probably fit on a ring, beam wirelessly to earbuds, and hold an infinite number of songs.

Oakley, makers of sunglasses and other eyewear products, has come out with an incredible new music player called Thumps, described as the world's first digital audio eyewear. This revolutionary new design integrates a music player and earphones right into the frame. You plug the sunglasses into your computer and download music into them. Basic control buttons are built into the frames and the attached earphones fit right over your ears. Thumps have the potential to hold an enormous amount of music, while eliminating the need for headphone cords and belt or arm straps. At present, they are not cheap, but they are a fantastic product for the runner who loves to listen to music. I received a pair as a gift from my wife and love them.

Music can be a very powerful motivator during run workouts. It can help you push through difficult training sessions, causing you to run harder and longer when your workout so dictates. I have created numerous music mixes for myself for use during different types of runs. Be careful if you decide to listen to music while running outdoors, however, especially on streets. Listen-

ing to music obviously lessens your ability to hear approaching cars and can decrease your awareness of your surroundings. You can easily zone out, potentially putting yourself in harm's way without ever being aware of it. Pull off at least one earphone whenever you are approaching a dangerous intersection and listen for any vehicles that may be near you.

ANTI-CHAFING PRODUCTS

As I discussed earlier, friction is one of the marathon runner's worst enemies. The farther we run, the more time surfaces have to rub against one another, and the greater the odds for major discomfort. In my experience, you can generally get away without using any anti-chafing products for runs of roughly two hours or less. Try doing a twenty-mile run without any lubrication, however, and you could be in for a rude awakening. The problem usually presents itself in the shower immediately following your first really long run. You are spent from hours of running and have been looking forward to a shower since mile fifteen. Leaning against the shower wall for support, you turn on the water and BAM! the water hits your body and you experience stinging like you have never felt before. Had you applied just a thin layer of skin lubricant in these places you would have enjoyed that shower rather than viewing it as some kind of medieval torture. A very popular anti-chafing product—and the one that I use—is called Bodyglide. This all-natural skin lubricant comes in a roll-on stick much like deodorant. When applied, it feels extremely light, non-greasy, and surprisingly dry—as if you haven't put anything on. Yet it provides a powerful invisible barrier that protects against friction. Some primary areas on the body where runners can experience friction include:

1. *Between the Thighs:* This includes the groin area for men and extends down the inner thighs for both men and women. This area is especially prone to rubbing because your thighs and running shorts can combine to produce major chafing. If you do not use a product like Bodyglide and you experience chafing in this region, it will often force you to negatively adjust your running form, slowing you down and even predisposing you to injury.

2. *Under Your Armpits:* This is an area you may not realize generates friction until it is too late. As you swing your arms back and forth with your normal running stride, they often rub against your sides in the process. Do this for three hours or more and you are bound to have some problems. By applying a light layer of lubricant on your sides you should be able to eliminate this friction altogether.

3. *Nipples (Men):* I am a member of the American Medical Athletic Association, and at a recent conference, a doctor presenting a lecture on friction used a term I had never heard before: the "red eleven." Many of you may not have heard this term either but know what it describes. It happens to runners who fail to cover or treat their nipples before a marathon and the simple rubbing of their shirts causes them to bleed. The blood then slowly trickles down the front of their shirts, forming a bright red "11" as a result. Stand at the finish line of any marathon and you will witness numerous red elevens passing by. Once again, this phenomenon need not occur with the most basic pre-run preparation. Before all your runs of thirteen miles or more, I recommend preparing your nipples for the experience. One way is to rub Bodyglide over them. You can also use Band-Aids, Breathe-Rights (designed for the nose but great on nipples), or liquid Band-Aid that hardens and provides a solid barrier against chafing.

4. *Sternum (Women):* Female clients have educated me to the fact that the sternum, underneath sports bras, is a friction hot spot. I would therefore advise female marathoners to apply lubricant to this area.

Applying lubricant to these areas should become a habit before all of your longer runs. Not only can chafing affect your LSD sessions, but it can also last for several days and compromise subsequent workouts as well.

Marathon Statistics

	2000	2001	2002	2003	2004	2005
Total Finishers	299,000	295,000	324,000	334,000	362,000	382,000
Percent Male	62.5%	62.1%	61.5%	60.9%	60.5%	60.0%
Percent Female	37.5%	37.9%	38.5%	39.1%	39.5%	40.0%

Source: www.marathonguide.com

COLD WEATHER GEAR

Because I live in the Northeast and train year-round, I do a fair amount of running in the cold. These runs frequently take place at 5 a.m. or 6 a.m., with no sunlight and stiff winds, so it can feel frigid. The good news is, if you dress properly, training in the cold does not have to be a particularly uncomfortable experience. Here are a few gear tips when running in a cold environment.

1. *Dress in Layers:* If there is one thing that makes training in winter more difficult, it's the ridiculous amount of laundry you will have to do when you dress appropriately. Layers are your friend when it's cold outside. The key is to dress in numerous layers rather than a single thick layer. Use performance fabrics as your base layers to keep warm and dry. I like my first layer to be tight, such as spandex shorts and a compression-type shirt, and I add on from there. Running tights or a thin pair of sweatpants (or both) may be worn on your lower body.

Note: A rule of thumb when running in low temperatures is that you want to be just a little bit cold when you first step outside. The reason is that your core body temperature will increase as you initiate exercise and, if you are toasty warm when you begin your run, chances are you will be burning up before too long. Of course, this depends on the individual, and you can always shed layers as needed. There is also that guy who runs shirtless when the temperature falls to the teens and below, but he's got other problems to deal with.

2. *Cover Those Extremities:* Your mom was right—you need to wear a winter hat when you venture out in the cold. As with other running clothing, there have been advances in the technical fabrics utilized in hats, so you don't have to wear one made of scratchy wool. There are numerous styles of thin and lightweight yet warm running hats that will keep in the heat, protect your ears from the cold, and absorb sweat efficiently. They are also quite compact and can be stuffed into a pocket or carried if needed. You must cover your hands as well. Mittens are a little better than gloves because your fingers will warm one another through skin-to-skin contact. Like your hat, gloves and mittens can be taken off and put back on as your body temperature and the outside temperature fluctuate.

3. *Wear a "Shell" to Protect Yourself from the Winter Wind:* There is often a fierce wind blowing during my early morning winter runs, and on those days I wear a "shell," or very thin running jacket designed to protect my upper body from the cold air. These fabrics are amazing; they are extremely lightweight yet provide incredible protection from the wind without making you overheat in the process.

4. *When in Doubt, Overdress:* There is nothing worse than going for a run in the dead of winter and being miserable because you are literally freezing your butt off. It is always better to overdress rather than underdress in these conditions; you can always remove your hat or gloves or tie a jacket or shirt around your waist. Also, if you want to shed layers but don't particularly want to carry them, you can always stash them in the woods or behind a wall and pick them up on your way back.

HYDRATION

In the past several years, there has been a great deal of debate concerning how to hydrate safely for marathons, and many of the old rules and beliefs have come under fire. This has served to confuse an already confusing issue even further. Much of this has to do with a condition called hyponatremia, which is a relatively new phenomenon at marathons.

HYPONATREMIA

Hyponatremia, a rare but potentially fatal condition, is essentially water intoxication. It is a disorder in your body's fluid-electrolyte balance that results in abnormally low plasma sodium concentration. Simply put, hyponatremia occurs when you do not have enough sodium in the fluid outside of your cells. When this sodium level drops, it causes water to seep into the cells in an attempt to balance the concentration of salt outside the cells. These cells then swell as a result of the excess water. This can pose a big problem for brain cells because, although most cells can accommodate this swelling, brain cells cannot; they are confined by the skull. Thus, many of the symptoms associated with hyponatremia, including nausea, vomiting, headache, and confusion, have to do with swelling of the brain. Several marathon runners have died as a result of hyponatremia in the past few years.

The bad news is that there is much conflicting opinion about how much and what to drink during a marathon. It seems that many runners experiencing severe hyponatremia had these characteristics:

- Excessive pre-race water consumption (often including the day before the race)

- Large amounts of water ingested on the course

- Slower marathon times (leading to more opportunity to drink water and sweat out sodium)

Note: On October 23, 2003, the Washington Post reported that hyponatremic runners drank as much as three quarts of fluid before the marathon and a pint or more at each water stop.

So what should runners do, given all the conflicting research, information, and advice? I recommend performing a simple sweat test. Weigh yourself naked, go out on a run of either thirty minutes or one hour without taking in any fluids, then weigh yourself naked immediately afterward. Your goal is to see how many pounds you lose per hour. If you run for thirty minutes, multiply the pounds lost by two to determine your hourly sweat rate. This will help you better determine your individual hydration needs. For example, when I performed this test, I found that I lost three pounds (I have a high sweat rate) during my hour-long workout. There are sixteen ounces in one pound, so I lost roughly forty-eight ounces of fluid in that hour.

3 pounds per hour x 16 ounces per pound = 48 ounces per hour lost

Therefore, I typically try to consume up to forty-eight ounces of fluid per hour. I believe in drinking every ten to fifteen minutes, so I would consume roughly six to eight ounces every ten minutes or ten to twelve ounces every fifteen minutes.

I have found one of the major problems with sports nutritionists' hydration recommendations is that they use measurements that are not very user-friendly, such as milliliters and pints. Who uses milliliters or pints when talking about drinking while running? Let's apply these amounts to real-world examples:

Standard-size water bottles generally hold twenty-one ounces of fluid; the larger versions hold twenty-eight ounces. If you plan on carrying these during training and your marathon, you can compute your needs accordingly.

You can find Gatorade Endurance Formula with the drinking top in convenience stores in twenty-four-ounce bottles. The regular formula comes in twenty- and thirty-two-ounce bottles. More on why I specifically choose Gatorade shortly.

It is obviously next to impossible to carry all your fluids during your longest training runs. Here are a few ways to ensure that you take in the necessary amount of fluids when there are no aid stations available:

1. Stash bottles at appropriate intervals along your long run route

2. Carry money and time your runs so you will pass by gas stations, convenience stores, home, or your car to refill your Fuel Belt or water bottles

Fuel Belts come with either seven-ounce or ten-ounce bottles, and the more popular belt holds four bottles. Thus, this belt should hydrate most people for an hour or so without having to refuel. Fuel Belt does make belts with even more bottles for those who wish to venture far away and be completely self-contained.

WATER OR SPORTS DRINK?

When we sweat, we not only lose water but electrolytes as well. Electrolytes include sodium, potassium, calcium, magnesium, chloride, phosphate, and bicarbonate. Research seems to indicate that sodium is the most important electrolyte for endurance athletes. This explains not only why the heavily researched Gatorade contains large amounts of sodium, but also why the company recently introduced Gatorade Endurance Formula with even more sodium. PowerBar recently came out with new PowerGels with additional sodium as well. Many top Ironman athletes carry sodium tablets on both the bike and the run portions of the race and consume significant amounts during their races and long workouts. Although the causes of cramping have numerous etiologies, a major belief is that it is often due to sodium loss through sweat. So, when it comes to hydration while running, my philosophy and strategy is based on the following thought process:

1. We need to replace fluids lost through sweat

2. We need to replace electrolytes, especially sodium, lost through sweat

3. Water contains no electrolytes

4. Sports drinks contain electrolytes, including sodium

5. We have limited energy stores and, in endurance events, need to take in additional energy

6. Carbohydrates are our body's preferred energy source

7. Water contains no carbohydrates

8. Sports drinks contain carbohydrates

9. Hyponatremia can be caused by diluting our body's blood sodium

10. Water contains no sodium

11. Sports drinks contain electrolytes, including sodium

12. Many top-performing endurance athletes rely on sports drinks

Why Gatorade? No, I am not sponsored by them. I specifically recommend Gatorade because it is simply the most heavily researched electrolyte beverage on the market today. The formulation is designed to optimally replace the things you need most in the least time possible with minimal stomach distress. The other beverages simply do not have this type of research behind them. This research continues to be carried out at the Gatorade Sports Science Institute, where extensive experimentation with top athletes is conducted.

Based on scientific research, anecdotal evidence, personal observation, and experience, I choose to drink Gatorade during my marathon training and races and recommend that you do the same. Given all the benefits that Gatorade-type beverages offer that water simply does not, there should not be a question about which one we ought to choose as runners.

Note: Many people complain that they do not care for the taste of Gatorade and therefore cannot drink it. Gatorade has heard this complaint over the years and now offers a huge variety of flavors from which to choose. Others complain that it is "too strong" and water it down as a result. This is a mistake; once again, decades of research have gone into Gatorade's developing the best solution both for rehydrating as fast as possible and for emptying the stomach as fast as possible. By watering down the beverage, you lessen Gatorade's effectiveness and should therefore refrain from doing so.

When it comes to eating and drinking for marathon success, here's my philosophy: Running a marathon is hard, and to run our best we may have to be slightly uncomfortable at times. This extends to eating and drinking things that don't taste perfect. You are not going out to enjoy a nice dinner; you are undertaking a significant challenge and fueling your body for optimum performance. Ideally, you should become accustomed to eating and drinking in training what will be provided to you at the aid stations. Because

Gatorade is one of the most effective sports drinks and also the electrolyte drink distributed at many marathons, it is in your best interest to learn to like it.

If you absolutely, positively cannot tolerate it, then you will have to find an alternative electrolyte solution. And as always, you will want to train with it and use it on race day.

It is a good idea to check ahead of time to find out which food and beverage sponsors will be at your marathon. You can often find this information on the marathon's website. You then need to determine which, if any, of these products you will use at the aid stations and what products you will carry, and then train accordingly.

I recommend drinking one to two cups of Gatorade or whatever electrolyte solution is on offer at marathon aid stations. If you reach a point when you can no longer tolerate the electrolyte drink, switch to water, then switch back if and when your stomach settles.

I believe a big part of marathon success comes from learning to run with the discomfort caused by fluid and fuel intake. In my experience, it is much easier to become accustomed to this than to try and perform well while dehydrated or energy-depleted.

HYDRATION GUIDELINES

Pre-run: Drink one glass of water or electrolyte beverage ten to fifteen minutes before your run.

During run: Drink an electrolyte solution every ten to fifteen minutes consisting of the amount in ounces determined by your personal sweat rate test.

Post-run: At the very least, drink a glass of water or electrolyte beverage after each run. I am a realist and understand that most of us, including myself, will not weigh ourselves naked before and after each run. Try it a few times, however, to get a reliable idea of how much weight you lose (these results will differ from your sweat test because you will be taking in fluids while you run). Current guidelines call for rehydrating with about sixteen to twenty ounces of fluid for each pound of weight lost.

Note: You may or may not have heard the term "salty sweater." These are runners who tend to lose more salt in their sweat than others. Salty sweaters often have white residue on their clothing after a run and can sometimes taste salt in the sweat running into their mouths. They may be more predisposed to cramping, especially in the heat. For these runners, electrolyte solutions that contain sodium may be even more important to performance.

2005 Marathon Finishing Times

Finish Time	Finishers	Percent
2:07:02–2:29:58	497	0.1%
2:30:00–2:59:59	5,741	1.5%
3:00:00–3:29:59	30,910	8.1%
3:30:00–3:59:59	72,942	19.0%
4:00:00–4:29:59	80,285	21.0%
4:30:00–5:59:59	73,307	19.1%
5:00:00–5:29:59	46,245	12.1%
5:30:00–5:59:59	29,751	7.8%
6:00:00–6:29:59	16,699	4.4%
6:30:00–6:59:59	12,001	3.1%
7:00:00–7:29:59	6,267	1.6%
7:30:00–7:59:59	3,996	1.0%
8:00:00–8:29:59	1,973	0.5%
8:30:00–8:59:59	1,185	0.3%
9:00:00+	1,212	0.3%

Source: www.marathonguide.com

Note: Recent research has indicated that caffeine and beverages containing caffeine cause no greater diuretic effect than does water during exercise.

NUTRITION

Just as there are questions surrounding appropriate hydration, there are various opinions and beliefs on whether food needs to be eaten during a marathon, and, if so, what types of food and how much. There is also the concept of carbohydrate-loading before marathons and whether or not this is necessary.

Simply put, I believe strongly in carbohydrate-loading and carbohydrate ingestion during marathons.

Carbohydrates are the marathon runner's preferred energy source. Protein doesn't provide a significant energy source, and fat would be great to use as our primary fuel because we have so much stored in our bodies, but unfortunately the body is not as efficient at converting fat to energy. The problem then becomes that because our bodies can store only a limited amount of these much-needed carbohydrates, when those stores are depleted, we quickly run into trouble.

Many coaches say you don't need to carbo-load or take in additional carbohydrates during your marathon as long as you eat a healthy diet. Let's be honest: The majority of Americans do not even come close to eating a well-balanced diet. Most people don't even know what a well-balanced diet consists of. It has also been my experience that runners who do eat well tend to take in fewer calories than they should every day. This is one reason they have relatively low body-fat percentages. They are strict about what they put into their bodies, they stick diligently to their workout schedules, and thus they are generally underfueled when it comes to marathon day. Here is a simple analogy: If your car gets twenty miles to the gallon and you need to drive 200 miles, would you put seven gallons in and expect to make it to your destination? By running constantly and restricting your calories without replacing them adequately, you are in essence doing the same thing.

Carbohydrates are stored as glycogen in your liver and muscles. They are converted to glucose, which is our primary fuel during marathon running. The average person stores roughly 300 to 400 grams of carbohydrates in the muscles and 100 grams in the liver. (Well-trained runners and those who carbohydrate-load can store considerably more.) Now for some simple math: One gram of carbohydrates equals four calories, so four calories multiplied by 500 grams equals 2,000 total stored calories. The average person burns roughly 600 calories per hour while running. So, if you took in no additional calories while running, you would essentially be "out of fuel" at approximately three hours and twenty minutes. This makes complete sense, doesn't it? Isn't this at the time when many marathoners hit mile twenty and bonk?

These numbers are actually on the conservative side of caloric expenditure; the more you weigh and/or the faster you run, the more calories you will burn each hour.

Note: If a 170-pound man runs for three hours at an eight-mile-per-hour pace, he will burn approximately 3,213 calories in that time frame.

These are all rough estimates, and there is a great deal of variability based on numerous factors. My basic point is this: I believe our fuel reserves need to be filled prior to our marathons, and we also need to fuel as we run.

Remember my story about hitting the wall during my first Boston Marathon? I believe that runners need never experience the wall if they do two simple things:

1. Fill up and maintain glycogen stores by consuming carbohydrates before and during the race.

2. Perform adequate training mileage, especially long runs.

If you do the math, it is no surprise that runners hit the wall due to energy depletion. It's all about energy stored minus energy burned, and we don't seem to be able to store enough to go 26.2 miles without nutritional planning and intervention.

So, as a marathon runner, consider carbohydrates your friend. This is not to say that we shouldn't take in protein as well as fats; we need those as well.

Carbohydrates: Our major energy source.

Fats: Our back-up energy source and additional fuel for lower-intensity workouts.

Protein: The building blocks for muscles.

There are specific times when each nutrient is called for, as explained below.

PRE-RUN FUELING

What should you eat before a run? Pre-race food choices are incredibly individualistic. Some elite athletes consume foods before their races that boggle the mind and go against scientific reason, yet they perform extremely well. Pre-run and pre-race nutrition is yet another aspect of your game plan that you must experiment with a great deal. You should keep strict notes in your running journal concerning what you ate, when you ate it, and how you felt and performed during your run. You must do this numerous times before you will begin to determine what works for you. And again, once you figure it out, stick with it. Determining your pre-run meal is especially important before your long training runs, because this will give you an idea of what will work on marathon day. Remember that a huge part of marathon success is mental and tied in to confidence; you will be much more confident the morning of your race if you consume a breakfast that you know has worked for you many times before. These little things make a huge difference and separate those who achieve their outcome goals from those who come up short.

Although you should experiment with numerous pre-run meals, food with carbohydrates as the main ingredient is where you should begin. You should also try to eat complex carbohydrates that will be released more slowly into your bloodstream. Good sources of carbohydrates include oatmeal, whole wheat toast with peanut butter, juices, energy gels, and fruit such as apples and bananas. You could also try the many types of energy bars such as PowerBars and Clif Bars for an excellent pre-run boost.

You must also experiment with how close to your run you take in food. I can eat as I'm running out the door and not feel any ill effects, but many people cannot. Obviously, if you get up early to run, it is not always possible to wake up an hour or two beforehand to eat. I think eating thirty minutes or so before workouts will do the trick for most runners.

Realize that breakfast is named that because you are, in effect, breaking an overnight fast. The liver might be fully depleted of its glycogen stores after a long overnight fast. Many people complain that they are not hungry in the morning and therefore do not want to eat before a run. Tough. You need to fuel up, even before shorter runs. Runners who are concerned with weight loss might not want to eat before a workout because they want to burn calories, not take them in. Research has shown that not eating before a workout can actually lead to decreased workout intensities and decreased length of workouts, thus leading to less net calories expended than for those who ate beforehand. Here, then, are the basic rules of pre-run nutrition:

1. Eat something before all runs, opting for carbohydrate-dense foods.

2. Experiment with a range of 25 to 50 grams of carbohydrates.

3. Keep fat and protein intake low.

4. Avoid foods high in fiber (to avoid unnecessary time in the bathroom).

5. Make good choices, including juice, bread, bagels, and low-fiber cereals.

6. Try to eat 30 to 60 minutes before your run, if possible.

7. Experiment, keep a journal and find what works for you and stick with it.

FUELING DURING RUNS

Many runners might not realize that an electrolyte beverage like Gatorade is not only great for fluid and sodium replacement but also contains carbohydrates for energy. Thus, by consuming a drink like this, you are simultaneously taking care of three crucial aspects of running success. As I discussed earlier, Gatorade has been extensively researched, and its 6 percent carbohydrate solution (fourteen grams per eight-ounce serving) has been repeatedly demonstrated to be the optimal percentage for speeding fluid and energy back into the body.

It is easier for your body to process fluids than solid foods, especially when you are running. You therefore want to try to take in energy in fluid form first, semi-solid second (think energy gels), and solid form last.

After extensive experimentation, I now drink roughly 8 to 12 ounces of Gatorade every fifteen minutes and take in a PowerGel (110 calories) every thirty minutes during my marathon races. My fluid intake will vary depending on the conditions, and my gel intake may increase at the later stages of the race if I experience any lightheadedness, but these intervals and amounts have become fairly routine.

I also try to take in PowerGels for runs of sixty minutes or longer. I therefore take one gel at thirty minutes for a run of one hour, at thirty minutes and one hour for runs of ninety minutes, and so on. The goal, as always, is to prepare your body for what your strategy will be during your race. What many newer runners don't realize is that the conditions of the race, including increased adrenaline and a faster sustained pace, can drastically affect the way in which your body reacts to taking in fuel. Thus, the more you can train your body to adapt to the exact feeding schedule you plan to use, the better.

Some people like to take in solid foods during their marathon. One technique is to cut up energy bars into small pieces and carry them. I recommend trying carbohydrate drinks such as Gatorade and gels first, and if those don't work for you, then by all means try solid foods. The bottom line is that you should use whatever carbohydrate intake works for you. Just remember that the more solid the food is, the more work it will be for your body to break it down and the longer it will take to convert it into fuel.

Post-Run Refueling

There is research out now pertaining to what is called the "metabolic window." This refers to the period of time after a workout when the body seems better able to replace fuel (glycogen) stores as well as repair exercise-damaged muscle (protein). In other words, you have a "window" of opportunity after your runs to take in nutrients that will help promote recovery from the workout and prepare you for your next run. It seems that the sooner you refuel the better, because this window closes after a certain amount of time. I recommend refueling within thirty minutes of your run. So what should you eat?

You can either eat or drink after your workout to refuel. The key is to consume carbohydrates and protein together; it seems that the protein assists your body in taking up the carbohydrates. There are numerous products on the market that are specially designed for post-workout refueling. Endurox is a popular recovery drink that comes in a powder form that you mix with water. It consists of a four-to-one ratio of carbohydrates to protein. In addition to helping restock carbohydrates and rebuild muscles with protein, Endurox contains antioxidants to reduce post-exercise muscle damage and glutamine to help reduce muscle stress.

Endurox Nutrition Facts

Serving Size:	2 Rounded Scoops (75g)
2 Scoops Makes	12 fl. oz.
Servings Per Container:	14
Amount Per Serving	% Daily Value*
Calories 270	
Calories From Fat 10	
Total Fat 1g	1%*
Saturated Fat 0g	0%
Cholesterol 10mg	3%
Total Carbohydrate 52g	17%*
Dietary Fiber 0g	0%
Sugars 40g	**
Protein 13g	
Vitamin C 470mg	780%
Vitamin E 400 I.U.	1330%
Calcium 100mg	10%
Magnesium 240mg	60%
Sodium 210mg	9%
Potassium 120mg	3%
L-Glutamine	420 mg

*Percent Daily Values are based on a 2,000 calorie diet.

**Daily values not established.

Source: www.endurox.com

PowerBar also makes a drink for post-workouts called PowerBar Recovery. It, too, is designed to replace carbohydrates and protein and is formulated with a ratio of approximately seven-to-one carbs to protein. Recovery comes in a powder form as well.

You can also make your own recovery fuel from real food. Peanut butter with an apple, half a tuna sandwich on wheat bread, a little pasta with chicken, and yes, even chocolate milk are all great carbohydrate and protein combinations that will aid in your post-workout recovery. I like to mix both strategies and use real food for some workouts, recovery drinks for others, and both food and drinks for my really hard sessions.

To use the car analogy one more time, you want to put premium fuel into your body rather than cheap unleaded. The better the fuel, the better the machine will perform. Carbohydrates are like "premium plus" fuel for marathoners, and we cannot perform to our fullest potential without them.

PowerBar Recovery Nutrition Facts

Serving Size	1 single-serve packet (45 g)	
Amount/Serving		%DV*
Calories	90	
Total Fat	0g	0%
Trans Fat	0g	
Sodium 250mg	250mg	10%
Potassium	10mg	0%
Total Carb	20g	7%
Sugars	10g	
Protein	3g	

*Percent Daily Values (DV) are based on a 2,000 calorie diet.

Estimated U.S. Marathon Finishers

1976	25,000
1980	120,000
1990	236,000
1995	312,000
2000	389,000
2001	366,000
2002	388,000
2003	400,000
2004	423,000

Source: www.marathonguide.com

CARBOHYDRATE-LOADING

There was a time when marathoners would severely decrease carbohydrate intake for three days or so, starting seven days before their race. And they would continue to train hard, further decreasing their glycogen stores. They would then consume increased amounts of carbohydrates for the final three days just prior to their marathon. This method was difficult to sustain, because training intensely while depleting your carbohydrate intake is not a pleasant experience. Further research revealed that this depletion phase was unnecessary.

Some who argue against additional carbohydrate-loading reason that if you taper correctly, you will burn fewer calories; therefore, if you do not change your regular eating habits, you will, in effect, be carbohydrate-loading.

Point taken, but I find this reasoning faulty on three accounts:

1. Many runners do not taper correctly and therefore continue to burn significant amounts of glycogen up until marathon day.

2. For those runners who may taper correctly, they still fail to eat an adequate diet rich in complex carbohydrates.

3. Even if you taper correctly and eat an adequate diet, you still need additional carbohydrates.

I can find no real downside to carbohydrate-loading other than psychosomatic issues. I have found great success taking in additional carbohydrates beginning several days out from the race, both personally and with numerous clients. That said, my definition of carbohydrate-loading does not mean eating one huge meal the night before the race. I actually would recommend against this practice. My strategy is to take in an additional 200 to 300 grams of carbohydrates for three full days prior to the marathon. I like to accomplish this through carbohydrate drinks, because I find this the easiest method. So, if the marathon is on

ately took several salt tablets and the cramping disappeared. This has happened on numerous occasions, so now I always race with a supply of salt tablets. Depending on the conditions, I might take in two salt tablets every thirty minutes or so. The moment I feel cramping, I take in an additional two tablets or more. I have run my best marathons utilizing this strategy. If you are a runner who fits several of the criteria listed above and tend to experience muscle cramps, you may wish to experiment with salt tablets both before and during your race.

Note: I will beat this point to death, but for good reason: Always practice for at least one workout what you plan to do on race day. When I first decided to use salt tablets, I put a bunch in the pocket of my Fuel Belt on marathon morning. This was the very first time I had done so. Well, as I've said, I sweat buckets while running, and when it came time for me to take a few salt tablets during the race, the belt was soaked through and the tablets had dissolved. I was literally forced to lick my fingers in a vain attempt to get whatever salt was left in the pocket into my system. If you plan on carrying salt tablets, you will need to find a protective container. A plastic bag, a plastic bottle, or anything that is small, lightweight, and easy to carry. I have two pockets on the back of my racing shirt that I use to hold a tube made by Fuel Belt for this exact purpose. Remember that whatever method you choose to use, you will be doing so under somewhat stressful conditions. You can always take in the tablets during a walk break, but try to make taking them as simple as possible.

SUPPLEMENTS

There are a seemingly infinite number of supplements on the market today. The dictionary defines supplementation as "something added to complete a thing, make up for a deficiency, or extend or strengthen the whole." We generally supplement to take in something that is missing from our diet, something we wish to have more of, or something extra that may bring about positive health effects. It can be overwhelming and frustrating to try to figure out which supplements you may need, what works, and what is pure hype. Running magazines are full of advertisements for the latest and greatest breakthrough products. The efficacy of these products can be quite suspect, and it is beyond the scope of this book to examine each supplement fully. I will tell you what I believe is beneficial and which supplements and vitamins may be a good start based on the latest solid research. I personally take the following:

1. *Multivitamin:* Some contend that you do not need a multivitamin because you can get all the vitamins through a balanced diet. Let's be honest: Even though runners generally eat a healthier diet than the average person, who can truthfully claim to eat everything he or she needs every day?

2. *Vitamins C and E:* Runners are more susceptible to free radical damage, an unfortunate by-product of aerobic metabolism. We can combat this by consuming foods rich in antioxidants and supplementing with vitamins as well. Vitamins C and E help fight free radicals.

3. *Glucosamine and Chondroitin:* There is great debate concerning the efficacy of these two substances. Glucosamine and chondroitin sulfate are found naturally in the body. Glucosamine, a form of amino sugar, is believed to play a role in cartilage formation and repair. Chondroitin sulfate is part of a large protein molecule that gives cartilage elasticity. Both of these may play a big role in protecting our joints and helping prevent osteoarthritis. Recent research suggests that not only can these two substances potentially prevent the breakdown of the cartilage in your joints, but they may also help in the formation of new cartilage. When the cartilage in the joints breaks down, it allows the bones to rub against each other, and pain results. Although the jury is still out on these substances, I am willing to invest in them just in case they do work. I do not have any joint pain, so I take glucosamine and chondroitin proactively. The brand that has been used in significant research, and the brand I use, is called Cosamin DS. It is not inexpensive, but if it works at all, it is a small price to pay in my opinion.

4. *Omega-3 Fats:* A "good" fat, omega-3s are found in certain fish as well as flaxseed products. Among their numerous suspected health benefits, omega-3 fats help curb inflammation, so they may help in the fight against arthritis. I am constantly trying new omega fat products; I have used Udo's Choice Oil Blend, a mix of omega-3s, 6s, and 9s, by adding it to my morning protein shake, as well as ProOmega, which comes in a capsule form.

Note: Be sure to check with your doctor before taking any new vitamin or supplement.

We should strive to get in all the nutrients we need through a healthy diet. But because this is not always possible and additional supplementation may prove beneficial, you should consider supplementing your diet based on your individual needs.

CAFFEINE

Caffeine is one of the most common **ergogenic aids** for endurance athletes in general and marathon runners in particular. In fact, caffeine is considered so powerful that the International Olympic Committee has banned it at certain levels. It is, however, perfectly legal for use by marathoners. It has several supposed benefits; the primary one for runners is that it may help our bodies use fat as a fuel, which can aid in preserving our carbohydrate stores and thereby allow us to run longer. The second major benefit is that it is a stimulant and therefore can provide a psychological edge. It can increase alertness and motivation, helping us "get up" for workouts and races. New research has shown that caffeine does not have the diuretic effect during exercise that it does at rest.

Ergogenic aid: Any substance or phenomenon that can improve athletic performance.

You should not overdo your caffeine intake, and for some people it may not have a positive effect. You can build up a tolerance to caffeine through habitual use, and its performance-enhancing effects seem to be strongest when it is used infrequently and primarily for competition.

If you drink coffee, a cup or two before your marathon may help with your performance. Like everything else, you need to try it during training to see how it affects you personally.

CHAPTER 4
Training

Yes, you can run a marathon after just sixteen weeks of training. With four months of training under your belt, you can also run a fast time if you wish, and you can remain injury free. To do so requires balance, however: not doing too much of any one thing but a little of several different things. And training can and should be fun. You should enjoy the journey as well as the destination. Training for a marathon is quite simply one of the best fitness goals you can set for yourself and, if you are disciplined in your efforts, you will arrive at the starting line looking and feeling better than you ever have before.

RUNNING FORM

A number of coaches and books claim to know the "perfect" way to run and that everyone should run using this one technique or method. I strongly disagree. Although I believe that many runners need to have their running form fine-tuned a bit, this often involves minor yet effective changes, not completely altering the way in which they run. We all have subtle differences in our gaits, and that is okay. Change this too much and injury might occur. I also believe that the more you run, especially the more long runs that you do, the better your form becomes. Why? Because I contend that the body is an incredibly intelligent machine. The more fatigued it becomes, the more it will adapt, getting rid of movements that are less efficient at moving you forward. That said, there are several common mistakes when it comes to running form:

1. *Swinging Your Arms Too Much Across Your Body:* You goal in running is to propel yourself forward, and if you swing your arms too much from side to side, you are wasting valuable energy. Picture an imaginary line down the center of your chest and do not let your hands cross that line as you run.

2. *Bouncing Too Much:* Again, you want to move yourself forward rather than up and down. Imagine you are running with a low ceiling above you, and keep the bouncing to a minimum. My sister-in-law Jen, a classically trained dancer who is extremely light on her feet, runs up and down rather than forward. Shortening her stride and increasing her cadence, or foot turnover, would probably help improve her form. For now, we just call her Tigger.

3. *Not Running Relaxed:* It may sound easy, but running completely relaxed can take years to achieve. There are numerous places where you can hold tension: your hands, face, shoulders, and neck are a few of the most common areas. You should periodically perform body checks as you run, going from head to toe to see whether you are holding tension in any part of your body.

   You can shrug your shoulders, bringing them up to your ears and back down again to release tension from your upper body. Shake out your arms at your sides every now and again. Bring your arms up over your head, interlace your fingers, and stretch your back and shoulders. Drop your ears to each shoulder to loosen up your neck. Twist gently to the right and then the left with your upper body to stretch out your lower back.

You can and should do all of these things while running, generally every fifteen minutes or so, to ensure that you are running as relaxed as possible. The more relaxed you are, the faster you will run. Something as seemingly insignificant as a tight lower back at the beginning of a marathon can rapidly become a major problem as the race progresses if you don't deal with it immediately. The secret is to do these body checks and perform these stretches before you have an issue, not in response to one.

RUN TRAINING

For those of you whose goal is simply to finish your marathon, you will just run. You should not be concerned with anything other than simply getting in the miles. It has been my experience that many runners benefit immensely from just running, without worrying about speed training, tempo work, or anything other than logging their weekly miles. The problem lies in the fact that many runners either do too much or too little, and both have negative consequences.

The first type of runner believes that "more is better"; such runners often over-train, with diminishing returns. They believe incorrectly that there is some nobility in training ridiculously hard. They read all the magazines and books on running and attempt to follow the training plans and advice that might apply to 5 percent of the running population, and these few are typically the professionals. These runners get hurt often and many become what I like to call "reluctant triathletes." Because they overtrain and eventually become injured, they are forced to cross-train in an effort to stay in shape while rehabilitating an injury. This often involves biking and swimming, hence a new triathlete is born.

There is an old story about a bee that was stuck inside a house and tried to get out. He was buzzing around a window, banging against it in an attempt to free himself. He would fly away from the window, turn around, then speed up and smash into it as hard as he could. With each failed attempt, he grew angrier, flying faster and banging harder into the window over and over again. What the bee failed to realize is that no matter how fast or how many times he hit the window, he would not achieve his goal, and that the window right next to the closed one was wide open.

"More is better" runners are like this bee. They incorrectly believe that running more, running harder, and running faster is better. They often leave their best performances in training and fall short on race day, if they even make it to the starting line. Many are forced to defer their marathon entries for the following year or choose a new marathon due to overuse injuries. Endurance running is a tricky endeavor to train for correctly. In life, great achievements are often the result of hard work, and the harder one works, the greater the rewards. This is not necessarily true when it comes to marathon running. As marathoners, we have a very interesting dilemma; we not only have to train to cover the long distance, but we also must be recovered enough on race day to cover this distance as fast as our goals require. This is why it is so important to train smarter rather than harder, and less is actually more when it comes to marathon training.

This does not mean that marathon runners do not have to put in the appropriate mileage; it means that it is the quality of training, not the quantity that counts. This brings us to the second problematic type of runner, the one who does too little. Less experienced runners start a program all fired up and with the best of intentions but soon start skipping runs and shortening or completely missing weekend long runs. They take the "less is more" approach too far and are not adequately prepared to run their marathon.

These runners rarely keep a running journal and are unaware of the gaps in their training. If you were to ask, they would tell you that they had followed so-and-so's training plan almost perfectly. They may not even be aware that their two supposed twenty-mile runs were actually sixteen and seventeen miles respectively because they ran by time and overestimated their pace.

It is the rare individual who picks the appropriate program for his or her abilities and goals and sticks with it. Marathon running success lies in three concepts: consistency, the correct program, and appropriate intensity.

1. *Consistency:* This means sticking with your program. Yes, life gets in the way, and no, no one is expected to get in 100 percent of scheduled workouts, but you cannot expect to run well if you have not put in the work. This means all the component parts: running, nutrition, hydration, strength training, and so on. As human beings, we tend to do what we like to do and avoid things that may be challenging or boring. We fail to work on our weaknesses, but it is only through practice and discipline that incredible results are achieved. None of these things needs to take a long time, either. You simply need to do a little

of everything consistently to achieve your goals. Think about it: By doing what you're not doing now and might not enjoy, you will inevitably bring about change for the better. Again, the body adapts to the stressors we impose upon it, and new stressors applied appropriately will bring about positive results.

Note: The definition of insanity is doing the same thing and expecting different results.

2. *Correct Program:* This refers to picking the appropriate marathon program for your current fitness level as well as for your goals. It is very difficult to create a hard-and-fast rule that will tell you which program of mine you should follow. People have such varied fitness backgrounds, fitness levels, and genetic makeups; I believe that there is no simple formula to determine which training program is best for you. Some first-timers may be ready and will benefit from running more mileage, while other runners may go faster by doing less. After finishing this book, you will be able to make an educated and, hopefully, objective decision as to which program is right for you. Much of this choice lies in setting a suitable goal. Marathon running is a

never-ending experimental process, and you will encounter many learning experiences along the way; this might also include which program you follow. Notice that I used the term "learning experiences" and not mistakes; these experiences only become mistakes if you fail to learn from them. You must constantly re-evaluate your training and results and tailor your program accordingly. It is always safer to start with the easier program and move up when you are ready, but the decision ultimately lies with you. Great things come from challenging ourselves, and I do not want to inhibit a great performance because of rigid guidelines.

3. *Appropriate Intensity:* If your goal is simply to finish your marathon, then you will run at a comfortable pace for all your workouts. Your goal is to build up your endurance so that you will have a great marathon experience and want to run another. Your pace will be the pace that is natural for you. The pace per mile is irrelevant; your pace is slow and steady.

If your goals are loftier than just finishing, then you need to add intensity to your workouts. They key is this: Where intensity is concerned, you will need to go hard on your hard days, easy on your easy days, and not spend much time in between. Many marathoners train in the so-called "gray zone," not running super fast, but not running particularly easy, either. There are often diminishing returns when marathoners train this way. These runners have no true long slow-distance, or LSD runs; instead of running slowly on their longer days, they try to run every workout the same way, regardless of distance. This is a mistake.

To run faster, you need to run easy most of the time and really hard a fraction of the time. This is especially true if you wish to have any longevity in the world of marathon running. Can you train really hard all the time and run a great marathon? Absolutely. If you continue to train that way, will you eventually become injured and have slower and slower marathon times? I guarantee it.

Successful marathon running is all about discipline: discipline in putting in the miles, in doing your strength training and watching your nutrition, and in running slowly when your workouts call for slower runs. If I were to identify one major training flaw in many marathon runners who want to hit challenging time goals, I'd say they do not run slowly enough on their easy days.

LSD runs are a perplexing concept for many. I believe you need to run these workouts at roughly one-and-a-half minutes per mile slower than your goal race pace. How can this be? How can you possibly be expected to run your marathon one-and-a-half minutes per mile faster than the pace you run during your long workouts?

You can and you will. These runs are meant to build up your endurance, not make you faster. There are five things that will allow you to run faster on race day:

1. Your shorter and harder workouts will give you the speed you need without running twenty miles or more at your race pace. They will also help improve your running economy, which is an essential component of running faster.

2. Your strength-training program will prepare your muscles to resist fatigue, improve your running economy, and hold the pace you need.

3. Hill workouts will add to your strength and allow you to run faster.

4. A true taper will provide the rest you need to absorb all of your training and arrive at the starting line rested and ready to run your best.

5. "Race Day Magic": There is probably no more powerful phenomenon than the effects of running in the marathon itself. The crowds, the competition, the adrenaline, the electricity in the air—all of these will be major factors in running the target race pace.

I believe in four basic types of run workouts: speed, strength, endurance, and recovery. Within these workouts there can be numerous subcategories as well. For instance, speed workouts can include track sessions, tempo runs, fartleks, interval work on the road, and shorter races. Strength sessions involve hill repeats of various lengths. Endurance runs are your weekend LSD workouts, and recovery runs are easy runs following hard speed and strength sessions.

Note: Should you run when you are sick? Many people use the "neck up" guideline: If you are sick from the neck up, it is okay to run; if you feel sick from the neck down, skip the running. You must listen to your body. Your goal is to be consistent; taking two days off from running is better than trying to run though it and ending up missing a week or more as a result. I often find that you can switch days and do your strength training in place of the run, because this will not tax your cardiovascular system in the same manner. Be smart. There are times when you will have to miss a workout or two due to illness. This is okay; no one gets in 100 percent of his or her workouts.

SPEED TRAINING

It may surprise you to find out that I am not a huge fan of doing speed work. Not in the least. Actually, it's not so much the speed work that I don't care for; it's going to the track that bothers me. There is nothing more painful—both mentally and physically—than running around and around a small oval at your **anaerobic** threshold. To be totally honest, I have spent very little time at the track and prefer to do my speed work on the road and at shorter races.

I believe that one of the main benefits of going to the track to do your speed work is the mental toughness that develops from these sessions. You will become faster because you are running faster, but you will also develop mental skills that will help immeasurably when you are being tested during your marathon. Do you have to go to the track to become faster? No. Running fast will make you fast, regardless of where you do it.

Many runners become injured as a direct consequence of doing speed work. Many running coaches state that if you want

to go faster, you need to train fast. Well, yes and no. My clients and I are living proof that you will get faster just by running, period. This is especially true with marathon running. If you want to get faster at the 100-yard dash, you need to train fast at 100 yards. But contrary to what many believe, you will get faster at the marathon distance just by logging miles. I believe that long runs are much more important than speed work sessions to most marathoners' success. Proper fueling is also much more important as well. I don't care how many times you sprint around a track; if you are not properly fueled and/or you did not get in your long runs, you will have problems during your marathon.

Never forget the Fifth Commandment of Marathoning:

"It is not about thee who goes out the fastest; it's about thee who slows down the least."

For those who will be following the advanced plans, your speed work intervals are outlined by minutes so that you can do them on roads, trails, and so on. If you really want to go to the track to do them, be my guest, but I would rather do them on the road, simulating what my actual marathon conditions will be.

My simple definition of speed work is running above your goal race pace for certain lengths of time. This can vary from running just above your intended race pace for ten minutes or more to performing shorter and harder anaerobic intervals.

Anaerobic: This literally means "without oxygen." If you cannot talk while you are running, you are in or approaching an anaerobic state. Runners will run in their anaerobic state or zone, during short-duration hard intervals to become faster runners. The majority of marathon training should be done in the aerobic zone.

One speed work session may entail running a ten-minute tempo at your 10K race pace, another may be five one-minute intervals at a hard effort with two-minute recovery breaks in between. I also schedule local races as speed work sessions. I will sometimes run just the race distance; other times I will get in additional miles by arriving early to run easy before and after. This is one of my favorite types of speed work sessions, the one I do most, and the one that I strongly recommend. An example would be if you had a ten-mile run scheduled and there was a 10K race nearby. You could get to the race early enough to register, and run two miles easy, timing it so that you finish just before the race begins. You would then run the 10K race hard, then turn around and run easy one

mile out from the finish and one mile back to cool down.

This is an example of great speed training in my opinion. This type of session has the added bonus of providing race conditions: the competition, the measured course, the aid stations, the pre-race anxiety, the adrenaline rush, and so on. The more you race, the better marathoner you will become. Race experience is something that only comes with more racing.

Marathon training generally consists of these types of speed workouts:

1. *Track Sessions:* You go to a measured track and perform "repeats" with recovery intervals in between. These repeats are generally one lap (400s), two laps (800s), or four laps (one mile).

2. *Tempo Runs:* There is much confusion about what a tempo pace should be. I like to think of it as a hard but sustainable pace. You're not quite happy to be running at this pace, but you can hold it for a decent amount of time, unlike repeats at the track. Think of tempo runs as being just outside your comfort zone. I consider these to be about your 10K pace, so you could, in effect, hold them for thirty minutes to one hour, depending on your speed per mile.

3. *Road Intervals:* This speed training is similar to track sessions in that you do harder intervals of five minutes or less, but you do them on the road within a run workout. For example, you may run easy for fifteen minutes to warm up, then run hard for five minutes and easy for two minutes, repeating this three times through, ending with an easy run for fifteen minutes to cool down. The shorter the interval, the harder you will run.

4. *Fartleks:* Swedish for "speed play," fartleks are essentially unstructured speed intervals. You spend a certain amount of time running hard to randomly chosen points, such as running hard to the mailbox, running easy to the telephone pole, running hard to the stop sign, and so on. Fartleks are a fun and easy way to add short speed sessions to a normal run. The day before your marathon, when you are running just a few minutes to get rid of your nervous energy, is a great time to throw in some fartleks.

Again, many coaches believe that to run fast, you absolutely, positively must train fast. Sure, if you want to run a 2:50 marathon, you will have to do speed work to train your body to hold that pace. But the marathon is an endurance event. Running a marathon is not only about going fast, but also it's about not slowing down. By simply running, you will train your muscles to be able to cover greater and greater distances with less and less fatigue. This is why I believe that slow long runs are actually more important than hard track workouts for most marathoners. Being able to hold your pace or even go faster for the second half of the marathon is not an easy feat for most, but with consistent run training, this can be accomplished.

LACTIC ACID

There is so much confusion and blatant misinformation about lactic acid and its role in exercise, especially when it comes to marathon running. And there is great debate among sports scientists concerning lactic acid and its supposed role in muscular fatigue. Essentially, your muscles constantly produce lactic acid as you run. What many fail to realize is that this lactic acid can actually be reused; it is a fuel and can be burned for energy. It is not all bad.

Your lactate threshold, or LT, is the point at which you are exercising at such a high intensity that your body can no longer clear the lactate from your system and it begins to build up. Some believe that this buildup, along with the hydrogen ions that come with it, may play a role in inhibiting muscular contractions, and therefore you must slow down. So what does this mean for marathoners? For the majority of runners, not a heck of a lot.

First of all, the only time your lactate threshold should be an issue is when you are running at high speeds and at high intensities, such as when you are doing speed work. If you are running at a comfortable pace or even slightly above it, you are not approaching or exceeding your LT, and it is therefore not a factor. Lactate threshold and the accompanying buildup of lactic acid have to do with anaerobic metabolism, when you are really pushing the intensity. This is not an issue for the majority of marathon runners. Yes, if you are doing speed work in training, you may be working at your LT or above. This is actually one of the goals of speed work. Research has indicated that by doing so, you push your lactate threshold back, meaning that the lactic acid accumulates at a higher intensity or a faster pace, and your body may also become better at clearing it at lower intensities as well. This supposed effect is one of the major reasons that runners engage in speed work. If this happens, you will be able to run faster.

For the vast majority of runners who go out and run at a comfortable pace, lactic acid should not be a concern. One of the most common falsehoods about lactic acid is that muscular soreness from running is the result of lactic acid. According to the latest research, this is simply not true. Many still cling to this belief, however, and arrange for a massage to help clear the lactic acid from their system and reduce the soreness it has caused the day after the race. Here are two problems with that logic:

1. Endurance running is done at intensities usually far below our LT thresholds, so this buildup should not even be an issue.

2. Studies have shown that generally two hours after exercise, our blood lactate concentrations have returned to resting levels. To re-emphasize: One to two hours following exercise, the lactic acid levels in your body have returned to normal. Therefore, how could the soreness after exercise, especially the following day, be attributable to lactic acid? According to the available science, it can't. The soreness is most likely due to the microscopic tears in your muscles caused by running, especially downhill running. This is why resting is so crucial to our success as runners; rest allows muscles to rebuild and heal themselves.

Finally, many runners attribute their slowed pace and/or their cramping during a marathon to lactic acid buildup. Unless they are running at an all-out sprint, they can't really use lactic acid as an excuse. Once again, they will undoubtedly be running at a pace far below their LT, so lactic acid cannot be the culprit. Glycogen depletion, dehydration, electrolyte depletion, or lack of proper training is much more likely to contribute to their decreased performance, not lactic acid.

For those of you who will be doing speed work and working your LT, I will have you run a cool-down after these hard efforts. Many runners who choose to end their workouts immediately after their hard effort and forego these final easy miles fail to realize that this cool-down serves a purpose. Studies have shown that lactic acid actually clears from your system faster if you engage in a low-level aerobic activity at the end of hard workouts rather than stopping abruptly. It seems the increased blood flow helps clear the lactic acid from the bloodstream at a greater rate.

So have your massage to loosen up your tight, sore muscles, but don't blame lactic acid. And definitely don't blame your bonk or marathon shuffle at the end of your race on it, either. If you follow the plans and advice in this book, you needn't experience either unfortunate condition.

TREADMILL TRAINING

I am frequently asked whether running on a treadmill is the same as running outside. I say, not unless the road where you live moves underneath you. All kidding aside, the short answer is yes, you can use the treadmill to train for your marathon. Many top professional marathoners do so and with good results. This does not mean that you should do the majority of your training on the treadmill, however. There are distinct differences between the two types of training, and, unless you plan to run your marathon on a treadmill, the more training you can do outside, the better. The more your training mimics the actual race conditions, the better. Differences other than the moving surface include:

1. It is slightly easier to hold a faster pace on the treadmill.

2. Many treadmills are actually at a slight downhill when set to 0 and are flat at 1.0.

3. You cannot control the hills outdoors. Unless you set the treadmill to "random," the terrain is entirely at your command.

4. Treadmills offer no uneven terrain or change in footing.

5. Treadmill running protects you from the elements, including sun, wind, rain,

and cold, conditions that increase the difficulty of your run and that you may encounter on race day.

Running indoors does have its advantages, however. It's obviously easier and safer to do so in extremely inclement weather. You can also control the speed and incline to your advantage for focused interval work. I also believe that running on a treadmill can help increase your mental toughness, especially if you do a few long runs on it. Running twenty miles on a treadmill is pure mental torture, but that kind of challenge can help make you a better runner. I encourage you to combine indoor and outdoor runs in your training to make you a more well-rounded runner both physically and mentally.

Note: If you choose to do a long run on the treadmill, I highly recommend watching a movie like *Braveheart*. I believe it's almost exactly three hours long (177 minutes) and will really make the time pass. If you are a real glutton for punishment and truly want to work on your mental game, try doing a long run on the treadmill with no outside stimulation whatsoever. No television, music, nothing.

MENTAL TRAINING

Years ago, running a mile in under four minutes was believed to be an impossibility. Many also believed that doing so could cause serious physical injury. Then along came Roger Bannister who, on May 6, 1954, became the first person to break the four-minute mile barrier. Although that was indeed an impressive feat, more noteworthy to me was what happened afterward.

Forty-six days later, Bannister's rival, John Landy, also broke the four-minute mile, beating Bannister's time in the process.

More than a dozen runners did the same within just a few years.

When people believed it could be done, they accomplished this seemingly unachievable goal.

Now I want you to do a quick experiment. If you close your eyes and imagine sucking on a lemon, really drinking in the lemon juice, what happens? Your mouth begins to water. Think about it; by simply imagining something, by consciously introducing a thought into your mind, you actually caused a physiological reaction in your body. That is pretty amazing. You can use this phenomenon to your advantage as a marathon runner. All of the best athletes do.

I contend that the top runners in any given race are all fairly equal physically. It is the one who wants to win more than all the others, the one who can and will suffer at the highest level, the one who directs all of his or her mental power to overcome temporary distress who will stand on the winner's podium. You too can use your mental powers to improve both your race performance and your race enjoyment.

The two types of mental training that are extremely beneficial to marathon runners are self-talk and visualization.

SELF-TALK

This refers to the internal monologues that play in our minds, the thoughts and conversations we have with ourselves. As the example of the lemon illustrated, these thoughts can have extremely powerful effects on the physical state of our bodies. Just think of the implications of being able to harness these thoughts to our advantage, to literally change the way we feel, to better our marathon performances. One of my favorite aspects of competition—especially endurance sports—is the mental game involved. Let's face it: The longer the race, the more time we have to think. So much hinges on your mind-set, on your mental state, and if you can learn to control your thoughts you can dramatically improve your running experience, both in practice and on race day.

You may think this whole topic is goofy and irrelevant, but you would be doing yourself a major disservice not to consider it seriously. You may be one of the many who thinks that the only thing you need to become a better runner is simply to run. Well, I hope you're one of the people I am competing against, because if you don't use mental techniques to better your performance, you've given me a major edge. Not to mention that I will most likely enjoy the experience much more as well.

You can use self-talk to do the following:

1. Create and change your mood.

2. Control your effort.

3. Improve your form.

4. Focus your attention.

You can quickly see how the ability to manipulate these four things can make a huge impact on your marathon performance. Running a marathon can generate enormous stress, especially as the race draws near, and mental techniques can help control these emotions.

I have a quote on the wall of my office that deals with the topic of stress. It was written by a guy named Lazarus and reads:

"Emotion is a direct manifestation of a person's appraisal of any given situation."

What does this mean? That a situation itself is not stressful; rather, it is our perception of a given situation that creates the subsequent emotions. In other words, it's all in your mind. The more control you have over your thoughts, the more you can control the way you feel. Literally. If you make use of the following mental tools, I guarantee that you will run faster and enjoy the marathon "journey" all the more.

CREATE AND CHANGE YOUR MOOD

Although you can use this type of self-talk anytime, both in training and in racing, it is critically important from the instant your eyes open on race morning. From that moment on, you need to play the following "mental tapes" over and over as you begin your pre-race preparations:

- "I am ready."
- "I feel great."
- "This is my day."

Self-talk consists of simple, positive statements, repeated over and over in your mind. You can use these or create your own, but they should start playing in your mind when your alarm clock goes off on marathon morning and continue until you cross the finish line. They can be sentences, song lyrics, or even single words—anything that will bring about a desired mood shift. So much can influence our moods on marathon day, including the weather, stomach distress, and injuries, and mastering self-talk to control your mood will have a profound effect on your race.

Just like everything else, you should practice self-talk during your training. On the day when you are running in the pouring rain, use self-talk to convince yourself how great you feel. Don't want to go out for that twenty-miler? Use it to change your mood and get out the door. Angry? Scared? Tired? Nervous? Overly excited? You can control and change any of these mood states by using self-talk.

I rely on certain song lyrics as self-talk to help alter my mood. I have created what I call my "mental MP3 player," and it has a specific marathon self-talk playlist. I selected some songs based on the lyrics, including James Brown's "I feel good . . . I knew that I would . . . So good, so good . . ." and Peter Frampton's "Do you . . . you . . . feel like I do . . ." I chose other songs for the music's ability to shift my mood. Both types are extremely powerful tools that have served me well in countless races. I also have a few isolated words that I use to change my mood, and I have linked each one to a certain visual that makes the effect that much more powerful.

Note: Many of you will wear MP3s and listen to music during your marathon and that will hopefully create and control the mood that you wish to achieve. Music is a very powerful tool in sports performance. Just think of all the professional and

Olympic athletes who listen to music just before they compete to get them in the right frame of mind. It doesn't matter whether your MP3 Player is real or imaginary; I just encourage you to harness the power of music. I happen to prefer my mental MP3 because it's lighter, it allows me to hear the cheers of the crowd, and the batteries never run out.

CONTROL YOUR EFFORT

The ability to control effort during a marathon is not a simple task, to say the least. I cannot count the number of runners who tell me, "I went out too fast," when explaining why they fell short of their goal. This goes for many veteran runners who simply cannot seem to hold back for the first few miles and get swept up in a pace well above their comfort zone. Go out too fast in a marathon and you will pay a costly price. These runners generally use the "on track" excuse to make them feel better about their lack of control. "At the halfway point, I was on track for a 3:30 marathon, but then [insert excuse here] and I finished in 4:10."

"I was on track for a 2:50 marathon at mile twenty when my quads totally cramped up. I ended up finishing in 3:25."

"At the half-marathon point, I was feeling awesome and was on track to set a per-

sonal best. Then I had some Powerade, felt like I was going to throw up, and had to walk the last six miles."

You must remember that a marathon is an endurance race. They don't give out medals at the halfway point, or mile twenty or twenty-five, for that matter. Using "on track" to describe your marathon performance is the equivalent of saying, "After the first ten questions on the SAT, I was on track for a perfect score . . ." Yeah, but there's more; that's the point. Always remember that a marathon race is 26.2 miles. Not one-tenth of a mile less. Use self-talk words or statements to hold yourself back at the earlier stages of your marathon:

- "Glide."

- "Nice and easy."

- "Flow."

I cannot emphasize enough how important it is to start out conservatively in a marathon, and these types of self-talk statements can make all the difference in the outcome of your race. It is extremely difficult to hold back when thousands upon thousands of runners all around you are going out way too fast. That's when mental tools become essential to sticking with your game plan. What makes pacing even more difficult early on is that numerous factors, including your adrenaline and the crowds, will make your pace seem much slower than it is. You will actually have to force yourself to hold a pace during the first miles that feels too slow, when in fact it is probably the exact pace you planned on running.

Self-talk statements are not just for slowing yourself down and holding yourself back; they can also be used when you need to pick up the intensity and the pace, such as when you're running up hills or sprinting to the finish:

- "Push it."
- "Pick it up."
- "Hammer."

Music and lyrics, whether recalled or playing on an MP3 player, can also be used to control effort. "Let it flow, let yourself go, slow and low, that is the tempo." These lyrics from a Beastie Boys song are among my favorite self-talk statements. This song falls into all four self-talk categories: It changes my mood, helps me control my effort, improves my form, and focuses my attention.

IMPROVE YOUR FORM

By using self-talk statements that involve process cues, we can help improve our running form. These are task-specific statements related to technique and may include:

1. "Relax the shoulders."
2. "Soft foot strike."
3. "Soft hands."
4. "Fast foot turnover."
5. "Relax the breathing."

These process cues are not only helpful in improving your form, but they can also fall into the fourth type of self-talk: focusing your attention.

FOCUS YOUR ATTENTION

This is one of the most important uses of self-talk as it relates to marathon runners: the ability to focus when we are in a state of distress. There will inevitably be moments throughout your race when you just don't feel great. Sometimes, it's minor; other times, it's major. You may have an upset stomach, an old injury might reappear, it may be too hot, your quads may cramp up—the list is endless. This is exactly when you would call upon self-talk to take your mind off the pain. You want to shift your focus away from the negative, and you can do so by using any of the first three types of self-talk.

For example, let's say I got a really bad "stitch," or cramp in my side, at mile ten. I would begin by immediately trying to switch my mood from a negative mind-set by thinking, "I feel great!" over and over again. I would then mix in self-talk that helps me control my effort to ensure that I am holding a reasonable pace while allowing the cramp to subside: "Slow and steady ... flow ... ." Next, process cues would take my mind off the side cramp while potentially helping to cure it: "Deep breaths ... Relax the breathing ... Relax the abs ... ." I would focus my attention by queuing up one of the motivational songs from my mental MP3 player and turning up the volume.

Finally, I would put a huge smile on my face. No matter how bad I feel during a marathon, I wear a smile. Oftentimes, the bigger my smile, the more pain I am in. But by putting that smile on my face, I instantaneously feel better physically. Try it the next time you don't feel particularly well during a run. Just smiling can work wonders.

So much of marathon running is about your mental state. Use self-talk to go faster and have more fun. It works.

VISUALIZATION

Top athletes spend a certain amount of time each week visualizing themselves having a great performance, and you should, too. Divers, gymnasts, skiers, golfers, you name the athlete; the best engage in mental workouts along with the physical ones. It doesn't take long, and absolutely it helps better your performance. Spending just a few minutes several times per week picturing yourself running a successful race has been proven to work. Some sports scientists think that visualization works because the human body cannot differentiate between what is real and what is imagined; in other words, if your mind "sees" yourself doing something, your body may believe it really happened.

All you need to do is spend a few minutes picturing yourself being successful in your marathon situation. I like to visualize the whole process, from the moment I wake up on race morning until I cross the finish line. You can perform your visualization exercises while you stretch. You can also do them wherever you wish; just find a quiet place, put yourself in a relaxed position, close your eyes, take a few deep breaths, and begin.

See yourself waking up and feeling great, no injuries, no stress; picture yourself walking around the staging area feeling confident and strong; see yourself standing in the start corral calm and relaxed; watch yourself start the race and hold your pace as people go out too fast around you; see yourself running effortlessly while holding your race pace; visualize the aid stations and how you will successfully take in your fluids and nutrition; envision yourself at mile twenty hammering past runners who have been reduced to the marathon shuffle; and finally, visualize your goal time on the clock as you cross that finish line with a huge smile on your face.

To be effective, like everything else in your training, you need to do your visualization exercises consistently. Not two times the week before your race, but several times a week throughout your entire training program.

When you do your visualization exercises, you want to make them seem as real as possible. The more you can do this, the more effective the visualization will be. To accomplish this, you must recruit all of your senses into the sessions: seeing, hearing, feeling, tasting, and smelling everything associated with your marathon. When you are visualizing, realize that you can do this from two points of view: either from your perspective (through your eyes) or from an outside point of view, as if someone were filming you. I recommend doing a little of both. As you visualize yourself running:

- See the sea of runners surrounding you.

- Feel the sun shining down on your skin.

- Hear thousands of feet slapping down all around you.

- Taste the orange Gatorade as you down a cup at an aid station.

- Smell the sweat.

The better you are at bringing in all of your senses and re-creating the true mara-thon experience in your mind, the better prepared you will be come race day. If you visualize consistently on race day, it will seem as if you have already run the course. This type of mental training will add a whole new dimension to your confidence level, and you will be way ahead before you even start your marathon.

REPLACEMENT

You will inevitably experience negative thoughts before and during your race. It is human nature, especially when we are exerting ourselves and feeling uncomfortable. When this happens, you should engage in a simple technique known as replacement. Like many of the other mental techniques, it may seem trivial and silly; but, just like those other techniques, it works.

So when a thought enters your head such as, "I hate this hill," you simply substitute "love" for "hate." As you pound up the incline, you tell yourself over and over, "I love this hill," and before you know it, your body will begin to believe you, and you will be at the top.

If your shins begin to hurt as you are running, and you're thinking, "My shins kill!" just replace "kill" with "feel great."

If you start to feel weak toward the latter stages of the marathon, and the thought

Boston Marathon Qualifying Times

AGE GROUP	MEN	WOMEN
18–34	3hrs 10min	3hrs 40min
35–39	3hrs 15min	3hrs 45min
40–44	3hrs 20min	3hrs 50min
45–49	3hrs 30min	4hrs 00min
50–54	3hrs 35min	4hrs 05min
55–59	3hrs 45min	4hrs 15min
60–64	4hrs 00min	4hrs 30min
65–69	4hrs 15min	4hrs 45min
70–74	4hrs 30min	5hrs 00min
75–79	4hrs 45min	5hrs 15min
80 and over	5hrs 00min	5hrs 30min

You can be 59 seconds above these times and still qualify. For example, a forty-year-old man can run 3 hours 20 minutes and 59 seconds and still qualify.   Source: www.bostonmarathon.org

"I am done" invades your mind, change "done" to "so strong."

Remember, what the mind perceives, the body believes. Control your thoughts to maximize your potential.

MASSAGE

Being a runner is a fantastic excuse to get regular massages. Running can make our muscles extremely tight and sore, and massage can help alleviate the discomfort. During hard training, I try to get at least one massage a week. To save money, I sometimes buy a package of thirty-minute sessions and have the massage therapist work solely on my legs. If I am really sore, I will sometimes book a full hour of legs-only massage. It is a good idea to get full-body massages too, because running tends to tighten your upper body, head, and neck as well.

Massage has two basic purposes for runners: first, to relax; and second, to help work out tight muscles. The first goal is usually at odds with the second, because loosening tight muscles tends to be rather painful and not terribly relaxing. Tell the massage therapist what to focus on based on what your body needs at the time. There is a time and place for both styles.

There are numerous supposed benefits of massage, some of which I support and some that leave me skeptical, but I believe that massage is absolutely beneficial for runners and improves performance. The taper is a great time to schedule a few massages. You will have been training hard for many weeks, and this is a perfect time to have someone help you relax and loosen your muscles. You can also use the massage sessions to practice your visualization.

ICE BATHS

Many top endurance athletes take ice baths after hard workouts. For runners, this can mean sitting in a tub filled with a few inches of freezing cold water, with or without ice cubes. If you saw the footage of P. Diddy training for the New York City Marathon, you saw him enduring an ice bath after a run. Although most people don't find an ice-cold bath the least bit enjoyable, research seems to indicate that it can help runners recover better and faster from workouts, especially hard ones. You can also fill a small garbage can with ice and freezing cold water and stand inside. Whether you choose the tub or can method, five to ten minutes should be enough time to soak and suffer. Try one after your next LSD run!

Note: Be careful if you choose the can method: When I first tried an ice bath, I filled a large plastic garbage can with freezing cold water and climbed in after a particularly grueling workout. Getting in required me to stand on a bench and slowly lower myself down. It took a few minutes but I finally got in; it was the getting out that proved to be exponentially more difficult. As I struggled to lift myself out of the can, I tipped it over, smashing onto my stone deck and bruising my hip in the process. I would therefore recommend using a much smaller can or the tub method; if you insist on using a big can, make sure you have a "spotter" nearby.

RUNNING CRAMPS

Believe it or not, the jury is still out on what causes cramps, or side stitches, when you run. What's interesting is that I used to experience cramps frequently as a beginner runner, but now I rarely, if ever, have them. I have found the same to be true with clients: Newer runners seem to experience these types of cramps much more often than veteran runners, who almost never have side cramps. This leads me to wonder whether there is perhaps a connection between side cramps and fitness levels or something else related to running experience. Other possible causes of side stitches that have been suggested include:

1. *Food or liquid:* What, how much, and when you eat or drink before and during a run.

2. *Inadequate warm-up:* Going out too hard too soon.

3. *Breathing patterns:* Too rapid or too shallow.

There are many other potential explanations, including one that contends that you are more prone to cramps if you tend to exhale when your right foot hits the ground. Why? Because your liver is on the right side of your body. If it is dropping while your diaphragm is rising, ligaments get stretched and may cause cramps. I'm not so sure about that one.

I believe that experience, pace, breathing patterns, and stomach contents are four of the best guesses as to what triggers side stitches. Since you cannot change your level of running experience, if you suffer from side cramps, I would focus on the other three possible causes.

1. Do not eat or drink too much or too close to your runs if side stitches are a problem. Also, see whether any one particular food or drink may be the culprit. This is why keeping a journal can be so important; you can record what you eat and drink and when you experience cramps to see whether there are obvious connections.

2. Make sure you warm up sufficiently. This may mean running a few easy miles before a hard speed workout or short race, or starting your runs at a lower intensity and gradually increasing the pace as you go. This is a good strategy regardless of whether or not you experience cramps.

3. Focus on your breathing and make sure you are taking in full breaths, not short and abbreviated ones.

If you do experience a side stitch during a run or race do the following:

1. Slow down.

2. Try to breathe deeply into the cramp.

3. Holding your stomach in can help. Tense your stomach muscles and perform an isometric hold while continuing to breathe deeply. This means holding in your abdominals in the same way you would tense up if someone were about to hit you in the stomach.

4. Use mental tools, including self-talk (see page 93), to focus your attention away from the discomfort.

5. If the cramp becomes unbearable, walk or even stop until the pain passes. Oftentimes, applying pressure to the area with your hand can help as well.

You can often run through a side stitch, especially if you are a more experienced runner. It may require that you slow your pace slightly, but side stitches often pass in just a few minutes.

BLACK TOENAILS

One of the unfortunate side effects of running a marathon or training for one is a black toenail or two. The black appearance is caused by the accumulation of dried blood underneath the nail. The cause is said to be the repeated trauma of the toe banging against the front of the shoe. For this reason, you should ensure that your shoes fit correctly and that your toenails are not too long. The blackened toenail should fall off after a period of time, and a new one will grow back. Although some people recommend draining the blood with a pin, I would leave it alone and let it run its course. It shouldn't be painful, nor should it affect your running in any way. Feel free to paint your other toenails black for consistency, if you are so inclined.

BLISTERS

Blisters are another rite of passage for the distance runner. Caused by friction, these small inconveniences can actually affect your running if they become severe. Your goal, therefore, is to minimize friction as much as possible. Make sure your shoes fit properly and don't wear thick, heavy socks. Don't run for extended periods of time in wet shoes, because this can lead to major blister formations. If you do get a blister, you can pop it and let the fluid drain, but do not remove the skin, which acts as a protective barrier. You can cover the area with a Band-Aid, if you wish. Rubbing an anti-chafing product such as Bodyglide or Vaseline on those areas of your feet where you are prone to blisters can help prevent their formation.

CHAPTER 5
Training Plans

The following training plans are all sixteen weeks in duration and include beginner, intermediate, and advanced plans. All have four days of running per week. Which should you choose? Beginners will run a maximum of thirty miles per week, intermediates will run forty, and advanced runners will do fifty. Beginners as well as those following the intermediate plan will just run without worrying about speed work, hill training, and so on. The advanced plan includes specific hill, speed, and tempo work for those who are more experienced and have higher goal aspirations. The choice is yours. I cannot say which one you should choose. Look at what you have done in the past and think about what your goals are—I believe the program that is right for you will reveal itself.

The plans are periodized, which means that the volume and intensity will increase and then decrease throughout the entire program. For the beginner and intermediate plans, only the weekly mileage changes; in

the advanced plan, there are also fluctuations in intensity. Periodization is an extremely important concept, especially the several "down" weeks when you run significantly fewer miles to allow your body to recover from the previous training and prepare for the upcoming training block. Runners who fail to periodize their marathon training risk injury, decreased performance, and overtraining. Remember: Less is more.

The plans incorporate three components of periodization: the macrocycle, the mesocycle, and the microcycle. The macrocycle for our purposes is the entire training plan, or sixteen weeks. The mesocycles I have designed are four weeks for base phase #1, three weeks for base phase #2, three weeks for the build phase, three weeks for the peak phase, and three weeks for the taper phase.

The microcycles are all one week in length, from Monday through Sunday, so your plan has sixteen microcycles within the macrocycle.

Sample 16-Week Periodized Marathon Training Plan

WEEK	Mon	Tues	Wed	Thurs	Fri	Sat	Sun
Base Phase #1							
16							
15							
14							
13							
Base Phase #2							
12							
11							
10							
Build Phase							
9							
8							
7							
Peak Phase							
6							
5							
4							
Taper Phase							
3							
2							
1							

See Appendix A on page 239 for 16-week marathon (and half-marathon) training plans for beginner, intermediate, and advanced levels. Note that the beginner plan increases mileage gradually and only contains one 20-mile run. The "down," or easy, weeks are week nine, week six, and the entire taper phase.

The intermediate plan increases mileage more rapidly and includes two 20-milers.

There are three runs of 20 miles in the advanced plans, plus significantly more mileage throughout. Down weeks include week thirteen, week ten, week seven, and the taper phase.

The down weeks prior to the taper are shaded a light gray in the training plans. Make sure you stick to the prescribed amount of running mileage and do not throw in any additional miles. These easier weeks are one of the keys to your success.

Yes, my training plans contain only four days of running. Although some argue that this is not enough for marathon training, especially if you want to run fast, I say, "Not true." The secret to success is not more; it is quality over quantity plus consistency.

$$\frac{Quality}{Quantity} + Consistency = Success$$

So much of endurance training is about avoiding injuries, and a big part of injury avoidance is rest. You don't get stronger or faster during your workouts; you become stronger when your body is resting. When we stress our muscles, we create microscopic tears, essentially breaking them down. When we provide them with adequate rest, they have a chance to rebuild and become stronger as a result. Many of the important positive physiological adaptations that we are seeking to achieve occur when our body is at rest. If we constantly break down muscle without allowing it time to rebuild, we will see diminishing returns and ultimately experience the **overtraining syndrome** and injury.

Overtraining syndrome The result of too much training combined with too little recovery time, the overtraining syndrome is characterized by decreased performance, elevated resting heart rate, crankiness, sickness, and decreased motivation.

By combining moderate amounts of running, resting, strength training, stretching, fueling, and refueling, you will run the best race of your life without injury. You will not do too much of any one thing, but rather a little of each every week. The problem is that we only do what we enjoy and leave the other things out. Doing too much of anything is not good for you, and this includes running. So often I hear about runners who were forced to pull back from their marathon training due to work, travel, family, or other reasons, and they ended up running the best race of their lives on less training. They also made time for things other than running, including strength training and stretching, and this contributed to their success. What is amazing is how many of these people fail to learn from this experience and go right back to running excessively and eliminating everything else. My goal and the goal for my clients is to run the best we can for the rest of our lives, injury free. Sure, you can run seven days a week, log insane mileage, and run a few great marathons, but that rhythm will inevitably be followed by injury, burnout, and a very limited marathon career.

My plans follow a simple formula. All levels run four days a week, but as the plans progress, so do the mileage and the specificity of the workouts. The weeks are broken down as follows:

Monday: Off. Rest day. This is necessary, because Sunday will be your long run day, so you have Monday to recover from the added mileage.

Tuesday: Run day and core workout. For the advanced plan, this is the speed day.

Wednesday: Strength training.

Thursday: Run day and core workout. For the advanced plan, this is the strength day with hill repeats.

Friday: Strength training.

Saturday: Run day. For the advanced plan, this is the tempo day. The tempo pace will be faster than your marathon goal pace.

Sunday: Run day. This is the LSD, or long slow distance, run day for all plans. Once again, it should be run at a pace approximately one-and-a-half minutes slower than your marathon goal pace.

One of the most common questions clients ask is whether they can move the schedule around due to conflicts, such as doing Saturday's tempo run on Friday and Friday's strength training on Saturday. The quick answer is yes. That is one of the benefits of running only four days per week; there is more built-in flexibility within this framework. Ideally, you will stick to the schedule whenever possible, but of course there will be times when you are busy on Sunday and need to flip Saturday's and Sunday's runs. It is almost impossible to do 100 percent of these workouts on the days prescribed. Your goal is to be as consistent as possible whenever possible. We are all busy and our lives are often chaotic, so you will miss runs and strength workouts. The key is to miss them only when truly necessary, not because you just don't feel like it. Consistency is crucial to your success.

Another common question is what to do if you miss a run. Should you make it up? The most critical weekly run is the Sunday LSD session, so if you miss this one, I would do it on Monday and stick to the schedule from Tuesday on.

If you miss a day, you can move that particular run or workout to the following day, except for Saturday's run. If you miss Saturday, just skip it, move on to Sunday, and keep with the plan. So, if you miss Tuesday's run, you can do it on Wednesday with your strength training. If you miss your strength training on Wednesday, you can do it on Thursday with your run, and so on.

Note: A common formula used to predict what your marathon time will be is to take your current half-marathon time, double it, and add ten minutes. Although this is obviously not 100 percent accurate, it is a fairly good estimate of your projected finishing time.

HEART RATE

I am going to get right to the point on this topic: I do not train by heart rate, nor do I consider its use essential to your running or marathon success. There, I said it. Sure, I own heart rate monitors—dozens, in fact—and heart rate is one of the many functions on my running watch. I frequently monitor my heart rate response during training runs and often record my heart rate during races. I do not choose to train by these parameters, however, and I have achieved what I consider pretty darn good results. It is my belief as well as my experience that the vast majority of runners really need not concern themselves with training within a certain heart rate range. Much more important is that they are consistent with their runs, con-

sistent with their stretching, consistent with their strength training, and consistent with their nutritional strategies. I believe in learning to determine how hard and how fast you are running first and foremost by feel. Heart rate zones can play a part in this, but for me, feel comes first. I know many of you hardcore runners and athletes will say that I am espousing nonsense; that especially for the more advanced runners, they must train by heart rate to maximize their results.

I believe that the primary benefit of a heart rate monitor for most runners is to ensure that they are going easy enough on their easy days. Most people think that the primary use is to make sure you are working really hard during those tough workouts, but I disagree. It's pretty easy to tell when you are running hard, but it's another matter entirely to run an LSD workout at your chosen slow pace. It's like the judge who was asked for his definition of pornography: He said he would know it when he saw it. The same holds true for your intensity when it comes to running fast: You'll know it when you feel it. It's the running slowly that you will most likely have a tough time doing at the correct intensity.

There are numerous problems involved with training by heart rate zones, including:

1. The formulas can often be highly inaccurate, underestimating as well as overestimating your personal zones.

2. There are many factors that can affect your heart rate from day to day, including, but not limited to, sickness, heat, hydration status, stress, and caffeine.

3. If you train outdoors and on varied terrain, it can be very difficult to stay within these often narrowly prescribed zones. Some coaches prescribe five or more heart rate zones, with some zones being just four to five beats from top to bottom. How can you effectively maintain these zones when you are confronted by such things as hills of varying grades and lengths, stop signs, and traffic lights?

That said, some of you will undoubtedly want to train with heart rate zones. If so, I highly recommend that you use a combination of **perceived exertion** along with heart rate.

Perceived exertion: How hard you feel you are working; your intensity level. I prefer to use a scale of 1 to 10, rather than the Borg scale of 1 to 20. Using my rating scale, 1 is the intensity of sitting on a couch while 10 is an all-out sprint.

For those of you following the beginner and intermediate plans, you will run without worrying about intensity. Your runs should all be between 5 and 8 on a scale of 1 to 10 as far as intensity is concerned, with the majority of your runs spent at around 6. When you climb hills or reach the end of longer runs, you will most likely move to a 7 or an 8 on this scale.

For those of using the advanced program, you will be doing speed work, hills, tempo, and LSD runs. On this same scale of 1 to 10, I would like you to maintain the following intensities:

Speed work: 9 to 10. These intervals will be relatively short, with none longer than 5 minutes. Begin the interval at an intensity of 9 and finish it at 10.

Hills: Begin the hills at an intensity of 7, accelerating up to 10 at the very end of the hill repeat.

Tempo: These should feel "comfortably hard." Because these last fifteen minutes or more, you cannot and do not want to run them at an all-out pace. You should run these at roughly your 10K pace, which I would equate with an 8 on the scale.

LSD runs: Most advanced runners have the hardest time maintaining the correct intensity during these workouts. I believe these should be run from one to one-and-a-half minutes slower than your goal marathon pace, erring on the side of slower rather than faster. You should run these at an intensity of 6 or 7, with the pace being comfortable throughout the workout.

There is a host of formulas that you can use to determine your heart rate zones. One of the most commonly used is the Age-Predicted Maximum Heart Rate formula:

$$220 - \text{Your Age} =$$
$$\text{Your Maximum Heart Rate (MHR)}$$

So, if you are fifty years old, your maximum heart rate would be:

$$220 - 50 = 170 \text{ MHR}$$

This is the formula found most often on treadmills, on gym posters, and in the calibration of many heart rate monitors. The problem, though, is that it can be highly inaccurate, either under- or overestimating a person's heart rate by up to ten beats or more. For example, I have a fifty-two-year-old client named Scott who frequently hits heart rates of 175 to 180 during his hard intervals or when doing hill repeats. He has frequently held his heart rate over 170 for fifteen-minute intervals, when, according

to this formula, that's simply not possible. I would even argue that Scott has more room to push his heart rate higher because he has registered readings of more than 180 beats per minute (BPM) on numerous occasions.

To determine your zones using this formula, multiply your MHR by the percentage at which you wish to work out. For most people, this is 60 to 85 percent for the bulk of their workouts, with hard intervals at slightly above these values. So for Scott, this would mean:

$$220 - 52 = 168 \text{ MHR}$$

$$168 \text{ MHR} \times .60 = 101 \text{ BPM}$$

$$168 \text{ MHR} \times .95 = 160 \text{ BPM}$$

If he were to work out at 60 to 95 percent of his MHR, he would have to stay between 101 and 160 BPM.

A second formula for calculating your heart rate zones that offers a greater degree of accuracy is the Karvonen formula. The Karvonen formula goes a step further and takes into account your resting heart rate (RHR) when determining your zones.

Note: The average person's RHR is between 60 and 80 BPM. Endurance-trained athletes will have lower values because their hearts become more efficient at pumping more blood with each contraction. Cyclist Lance Armstrong reportedly has a RHR of approximately 33 BPM and a maximum heart rate of 201 BPM. Once again, using the Age-Predicted Maximum Heart Rate formula, Lance's maximum heart rate translates to that of a nineteen-year-old.

The best way to determine your personal resting heart rate is to take it first thing in the morning, just after you wake up. You can use your heart rate monitor or a watch, counting the number of heart beats in a minute or the number of beats in a fifteen-second interval and multiplying by four. You should do this for three mornings and take an average of the three readings to find your RHR.

KARVONEN FORMULA

220 – Your Age = MHR – RHR x % of heart rate you wish to train at + RHR

You subtract your RHR from your MHR, multiply it by the percentage of your MHR at which you wish to train, and then add your RHR back in to arrive at this value. Let's use Scott again as an example and compare the two results. He has a RHR of

53, and he is 52 years old. First, we will determine what 60 percent of his MHR would be using the Karvonen formula and then what 95 percent would be:

$$220 - 52 = 168 - 53 = 115 \times .60$$
$$= 69 + 53 = 122 \text{ BPM}$$

$$220 - 52 = 168 - 53 = 115 \times .95$$
$$= 109 + 53 = 162 \text{ BPM}$$

For Scott, using the Karvonen formula, his zones for 60 to 95 percent would be 122 to 162 BPM. Let's compare that to the Age-Predicted Heart Rate zones:

Age-Predicted Heart Rate Zones:
60% to 95% = 101 to 160 BPM

Karvonen Heart Rate Zones:
60% to 95% = 122 to 162 BPM

Rather than using these types of formulas alone (and there are indeed many more than these two), I prefer to get heart rate data using "field tests," namely races. The client wears his or her heart rate monitor during several 5K and 10K races, and we note the average heart rates as well as the MHRs. This is not enough in my experience. I also have clients wear their heart rate monitors during the different runs each week for several weeks and record that data, too. Then, taking all this information into account, I structure several different heart rate zones for them based on their training and racing history. Determining heart rate zones is a lengthy process and can include significant variability. Throw in additional variables such as heat, stress, cardiovascular drift, which is related to reduced maximal oxygen uptake during heat stress, and caffeine, and matters become even more complicated.

If you must train by heart rate zones, I encourage you to use the Karvonen formula and monitor your heart rate during 5K and 10K races. I would then apply them to my plan as follows:

Tuesdays: Run intervals at 90 to 100 percent, beginning at the lower end and gradually increasing the intensity. This should approximately be your 5K pace or faster.

Thursdays: Run the hills hard, from 80 to 100 percent, beginning at the lower end and gradually increasing the intensity.

Saturdays: Run the tempos at 80 to 90 percent, trying to maintain a steady state throughout. This should approximately be your 10K pace.

Sundays: Easy. Try to hold the entire run from 60 to 75 percent, trying to maintain a steady state throughout. This should be around one to one-and-a-half minutes slower than your marathon goal pace.

For the warm-up and cool-down miles on Tuesdays, Thursdays, and Saturdays, warm up at 60 percent and gradually increase to 80 percent before the work intervals. Cool down slowly, bringing the heart rate and pace down gradually after the work intervals, until at the end of the workout you are around 60 percent.

Let me end by saying that the overriding benefit of heart rate monitoring for the vast majority of runners is its usefulness as training data rather than as a strict parameter in which to train. We know we are getting fitter when we can maintain the same pace at a lower heart rate. In other words, if you run a 10K race averaging seven-minute miles at a heart rate of 150, and weeks later you run another 10K race averaging seven-minute miles at an average heart rate of 145, then you have made definite progress. If you do hill repeats one week and your MHR averages out at 170, and then weeks later it's down to 163 on the same hill, that's a good sign. Also, one of the greatest uses of heart rate data is to see how fast you recover from a hard interval. The fitter you are, the faster your heart rate will drop. Once again, when you are doing your hill repeats, if you choose to use a monitor, notice what your heart rate is at the bottom of the hill after a repeat. Your heart rate should be lower before each successive hill repeat as you increase your level of fitness.

If you choose to use a heart rate monitor, I therefore encourage you to use it as a data-gathering device rather than as the sole determinant of the structure of your workouts. Learn to go by feel, and use a heart rate monitor to help you increase your level of body awareness.

STRENGTH TRAINING

To lift weights or not to lift weights, that is the question. There are many "experts" who say that marathon runners should not lift weights at all. Some contend that strength training does not help runners in any measurable way. Others go a step further, saying not only that lifting weights will not make you a better runner, but also that it will actually slow you down.

I believe both groups are wrong.

Many of these same experts also insist that time spent doing anything other than running is a waste of time.

Yes, there is something called the S.A.I.D. principle in exercise, an acronym for Specific Adaptations to Imposed Demands, which suggests that you get better at something by designing your training as closely as possible to that which you wish to improve. In other words, if you want to become better at running hills, then you should run hills. Makes sense, but does this mean that you should just run hills? I don't think so.

One of the biggest problems with sports science is whether the findings in the studies can be applied to real-world situations. Suppose, for instance, there is a study that examines whether strength training improves running endurance. After the experiment is concluded, the researchers state that no, their data shows that strength training does not improve running endurance. They release their paper, the media pick it up, and soon there are headlines everywhere that declare: "Strength Training Does Not Improve Marathon Performance." Well, there are so many variables involved that I have a hard time making the huge leap to the conclusions that many draw from these types of studies. What was the prior training level of the participants? What were the exercises used in the study? How long was the study? How many sets and repetitions were specified? How much weight did the participants lift? How many times per week? And so on. Once again, in both my personal experience and my experience training thousands of clients, I have found strength training to be an essential component of long-term running success. Like everything else in fitness and exercise, there are innumerable studies that support both sides of the argument.

It has also been my experience that the coaches who do not believe in strength training have an inordinately higher percentage of injured runners and "accidental triathletes." My goal is to run well into my later years, and to do this I must remain injury free. Sure, you can set a few marathon PRs in your early years by logging extremely high mileage, avoiding strength training, and pushing the speed-work envelope, but you will probably pay a heavy price.

I believe that the number one reason marathoners should strength train is injury prevention. As I stated earlier, I believe that running does not cause injuries; it merely illuminates our weak links. Strength training is one of the primary means by which we can strengthen and ultimately eliminate these weaknesses, which manifest themselves in three main ways:

1. *Muscular Imbalances:* Some of us have muscular imbalances to begin with, some create these imbalances through running, and many have a combination of both. By implementing targeted strength training, we can help fix these problems.

2. *Muscular Weaknesses:* Many people have dramatic muscular weaknesses, and this is why so many people state that they can't run. It is also one of the main reasons those who do run eventually end up injured. Knee issues, hip issues, back issues—much of the pain that presents itself after running can be alleviated by intelligent strength work.

3. *Individual Biomechanical Differences:* We are, in fact, not all created equal. Our bodies are vastly different from one another, and these differences can lead to problems. Leg-length discrepancies, quadriceps angles, and our personal running gaits can create issues that can be addressed through resistance training.

I contend that strength training also improves running strength, running endurance, and running economy. In particular, I believe that **plyometric** drills and **unilateral** exercises are invaluable to the runner for performance and injury prevention.

Plyometrics: Jumping and bounding exercises that involve repeated rapid stretching and contracting of muscles to increase muscle strength and power. Jumping onto a box is an example of a plyometric exercise.

Unilateral exercise: Using one side of the body at a time. Single-leg ball squats are an example of a unilateral exercise.

THE CORE

Core training is a part of my strength workouts and is another essential component of a well-balanced training plan. The definition of the "core" musculature may vary slightly from one fitness professional to another. For our purposes, the core consists of the abdominal muscles and the muscles of the lower back: the front and back of your midsection. Having a strong core helps prevent injury and improves performance.

A weak core means a decreased running economy and therefore slower times. Think about it: If the middle of your body is weak or imbalanced, it will greatly affect your overall strength and stability. It can also lead to abnormalities in your running gait, which can result in injury. The great news about core work is that it is simple to do, it requires almost no equipment, and each session need last only five to ten minutes. Once again, it is consistency that makes all the difference when it comes to strengthening your core.

Each plan contains core work. As the plans progress, the core work becomes more involved. The core work is simple, and a little goes a long way. You will do core workouts every Tuesday and Thursday within your strength program, and you will do one additional core workout on Saturday as well.

PRINCIPLES OF SUCCESSFUL STRENGTH TRAINING

Having spent more than two decades in the gym training myself and my clients, I have learned five basic principles that bring about major success:

1. *Focus on Form:* When it comes to lifting weights, maintaining proper form is crucial. I always say that squats and lunges are not bad for you; bad squats and bad lunges can be bad for you. Unfortunately, this can be extremely confusing because many so-called "fitness professionals" use poor form when they perform exercises. Use the pictures in this book to see how to position your body. Read the exercise descriptions and follow the instructions. Also, make use of a mirror at home or at the gym whenever possible when performing your exercises. This is not about vanity; it's to ensure that your body is properly aligned throughout the entire range of motion. We are born with different levels of "kinesthetic awareness," which is basically an awareness of our body's position in space. Some people, such as gymnasts and divers, have much better

kinesthetic awareness than others. Using proper form will bring about greater results from your strength work and prevent potential injury.

2. *Choose the Appropriate Weight:* Generally speaking, men lift weights that are too heavy and women lift weights that are too light. Both training errors lead to poor results and possible injury. An incorrect weight selection is, in my opinion, a primary reason why people do not achieve their objectives from their weight-training programs. You must choose a weight that makes the last few repetitions challenging while allowing you to maintain proper form. This is extremely important. There is a concept known as the "overload principle." It basically means that you must challenge or "overload" your muscles to bring about positive change. When you use weights that are too heavy, you end up using momentum and muscles other than the ones you wish to target. When the weight is too light, you do not adequately overload the muscle and the results are therefore diminished.

One problem with choosing the appropriate weight is that it will take time to determine the exact poundage for each exercise. This is to be expected and is another reason you must stick with your program and not look for immediate results. A major benefit of my strength-training programs is that they require little additional weight other than your body weight. Over time, you may add weight to these exercises, perhaps by holding dumbbells for squats and lunges, as long as you don't compromise your form in the process. You can achieve great results without additional weight by paying strict attention to the speed at which you perform each exercise, which leads to the next principle: "Slow It Down."

3. *Slow It Down:* Once you have selected the appropriate weight, implementing this principle becomes paramount to your success. Slowing it down means taking your time to perform each repetition. This generally means taking roughly two seconds to raise the weight, and, more important, three to four seconds to lower the weight. Most people completely ignore the lowering of the weight, letting gravity or momentum do all the work, and this greatly reduces the effectiveness of the exercise. Take a squat, for example: You should lower your body to the ground slowly, keeping the tension in your leg muscles during the entire descent. You then raise your body

up a little faster than it took you to go down, pause for a moment, and then slowly begin to lower yourself back down again. By engaging the muscle with "time under tension," you will bring about the changes you hope to achieve. Push ups, crunches, you name it; slow all these exercises down and focus on the muscle that you are working. This is why weight selection is so crucial; if you choose a weight that is too heavy, you will be unable to control it adequately. This, in turn, will make you perform each repetition faster than you should in order to move the weight, thereby losing the effectiveness of the exercise and setting you up for injury. Slower is always better. Avoid using additional weights for body weight exercises (lunges, squats, step ups); focus instead on slowing it down until you are really ready to make the exercise more challenging.

4. *Work on Your Weaknesses:* Here is a commonsense principle that is so rarely implemented. As human beings, we tend to do what we excel at and what we enjoy, with the result that we do not improve and we create imbalances that can lead to injury. Running is tremendous at illuminating our individual weaknesses. If we do not

address these issues immediately, at the first signs of trouble, they can become injuries that may force us to stop running altogether. Do the exercises that you least enjoy at the beginning of each workout. Get them out of the way right away. You will be amazed at how much you improve by allocating just a few minutes each session to the exercises that you would rather skip. For example, I'm not a big fan of doing exercises to strengthen my lower back, but I know how crucial a strong back is to running longevity. Doing two sets of an exercise such as back extensions is so easy and takes so little time, yet it can make such a huge difference in the long run (pun intended).

5. *Be Proactive, Not Reactive:* Let's face it: So much of what most runners do other than running is reacting to a problem. Physical therapy, stretching, icing, specific strength work, acupuncture, massage—most of these are undertaken after a problem has arisen. If you follow the steps outlined in this book and apply the concepts consistently, you will have to react to these types of problems much less frequently. And if the problems do arise, you will be able to solve them much faster as well. This is why full-body workouts are so essential. Don't wait until you have

back problems to strengthen your core; work on your core while you are healthy. Don't wait to strengthen your shins until you have issues with your lower legs; do toe raises now to strengthen your anterior tibialis muscles (shins). We want to run injury free for the rest of our lives and, by being proactive in our strength training, we can make that possible.

6. *Just Do It—Consistently:* If I've learned anything over the years as a coach and an athlete, it's that consistency is key. True success does not come from doing anything occasionally, such as occasionally stretching for thirty minutes, occasionally refueling after a hard workout, or occasionally lifting weights. Success comes from doing the basics consistently. It comes from having a strength-training plan and following that plan. Not doing more, not doing less, but just doing it week in and week out. Many runners fool themselves and believe that strength training doesn't help because they engage in a few sessions with no discernible results. They tend to overestimate the number of times they did their strength-training workout when, in fact, they had major gaps in their program. Life will of course get in the way, and you will miss a workout here and there, but if you make consistency a priority, you will reap huge rewards.

One major note about strength training and running: When you first engage in strength training and for some time after, your runs will most likely be affected. Your legs will feel like lead and you will run slower. This is another reason many runners do not strength train. They try it and, when they cannot go out and run as fast as they want to, they drop it altogether.

You need to focus on your race goal. How fast you run during training is not as important as how strong and how prepared you are for your marathon. You may be sore after these workouts and you will run a little slower as a result, but if you stick with it and taper correctly, you will not only avoid injury, but you will also run faster on race day. This takes a great deal of faith and means that you may run a little more slowly than you care to in shorter training races.

Ego

A tremendous amount of running success comes from delayed gratification as well as from keeping our egos in check while training. This means that you must stick to your workout at all times and not turn a Sunday LSD run into an interval session just because a runner, whom you believe you are faster than, sprints by you and you must keep up with him. I cannot tell you how many athletes I have seen who leave it all in practice and have mediocre races because they let their egos get the best of them during training. Many also get hurt by turning what is supposed to be an easy run into a speed session because of other runners around them. Do you want to beat that aforementioned runner, who probably is just going out for a two-mile run while you are on your fourteenth mile, or do you want to have a great marathon performance? This goes for training races, too. If you are using a training race as a workout and have a specific pace you need to keep, don't push that pace just to beat other runners. This takes discipline, and if you can learn it during training, you will be able to use it at the most crucial time—during the early miles of your marathon when almost everyone is running too fast.

You should choose your strength-training plan based on your fitness level, weight-training experience, race goals, and availability of equipment. The Beginner Plan and Intermediate Plan A can both be done entirely at home with minimal equipment. For those who wish to follow the Intermediate Plan B and the Advanced Plan, you will need access to a gym.

Beginner Plan—13 weeks

Exercise	Sets	Reps	Notes
Push up	3	to failure	Beginners may start on knees and progress to full push ups. Lower slowly until your chest is a few inches off the floor, then return to starting position. See photos page 122.
Dumbbell row	2	12 each arm	Bend at the waist, leaning forward with one elbow resting on your knee and your opposite leg extended behind you. Position your upper body so it is parallel to the floor and the natural curve remains in your lower back. Begin with your arm extended down toward the floor; raise the weight up toward your armpit. Hold for 1 second and lower. See photos page 123.
Squat (dumbbells optional)	2	15	Stand with your feet a little wider than shoulder-width. See photos page 124 and 125.

Stationary lunge (dumbbells optional)	2	10 each leg	Stand in a split stance with one leg forward and one back. Keeping your chest up and your knee behind your toes, lower your body straight down to the floor until your back knee is almost touching the floor. Hold for 1 second, then return to starting position. See photos page 126 and 127.

Core Exercises

Regular crunch	2	20	Lie on the floor with your knees bent and your hands folded across your chest. Keeping your chin off your chest, slowly lift your upper body off the floor, hold for 1 second, then lower back down. See photos page 128.
Oblique crunch	2	15 each side	Lie on the floor with one knee bent up and the other leg crossed with the ankle resting on the thigh. Place the hand on the same side of the body as the bent leg behind your head, and bring that elbow toward your raised knee while twisting and bringing that shoulder blade off the floor. Lower down but do not allow the shoulder blade to touch the floor for the remainder of the exercise. See photos page 129.
Plank	1	30 seconds	Assume a push-up position but support your upper body on your forearms and press your palms together. Keep your body perfectly straight and abdominals tight while breathing normally. Hold for 1 minute or until you lose your form. If your form fails early, you may rest on your knees for a few seconds, then return to plank and hold, repeating for one minute. The goal is a 60-second hold. See photos page 130.
Superman	2	10	Lie on your stomach with your arms straight above your head. Simultaneously lift both hands and feet off the floor, squeezing the muscles of your lower back. Hold for 1 second, then slowly lower. See photos page 130.

Push up

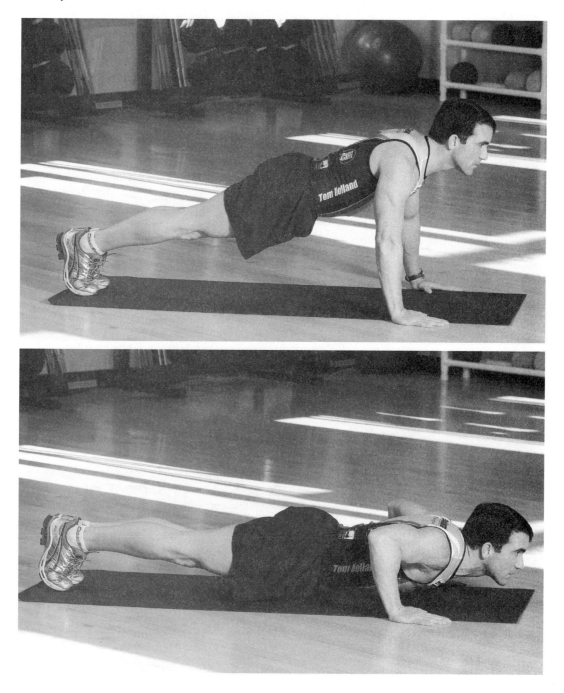

Dumbbell row

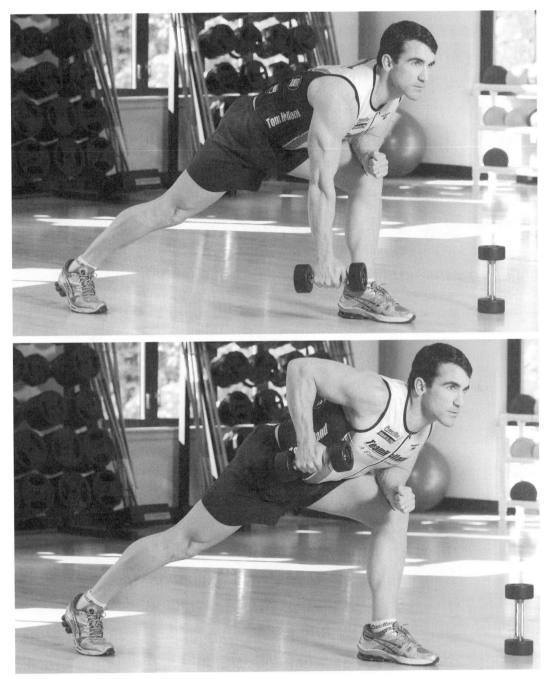

Squat
(dumbbells optional)

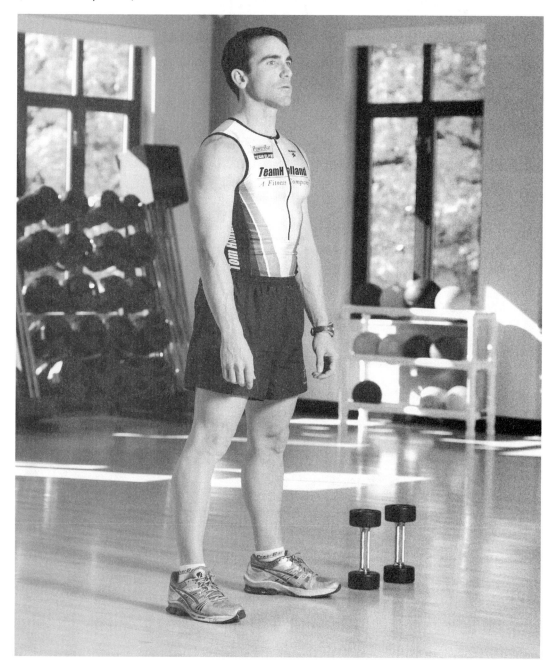

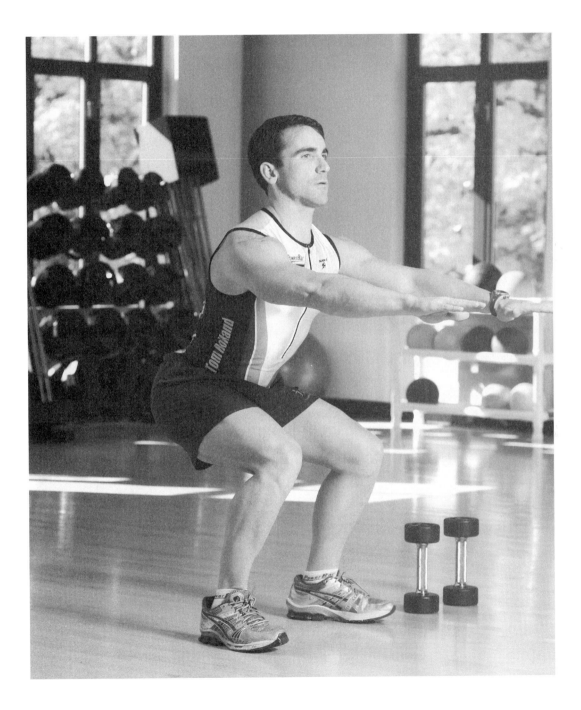

Stationary lunge

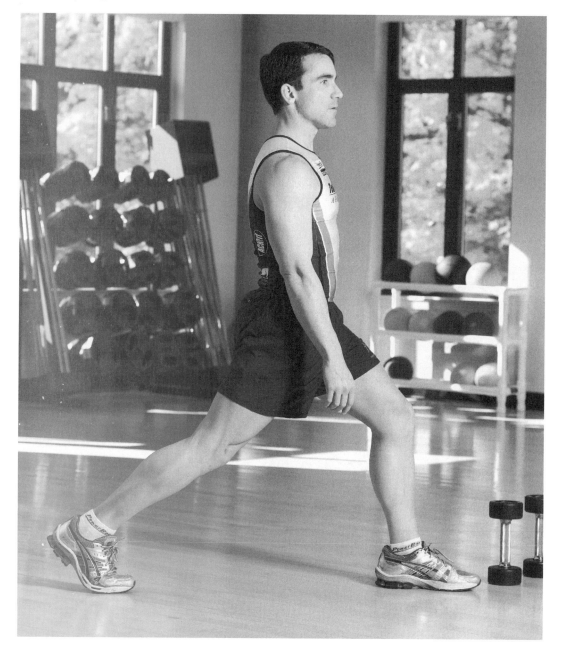

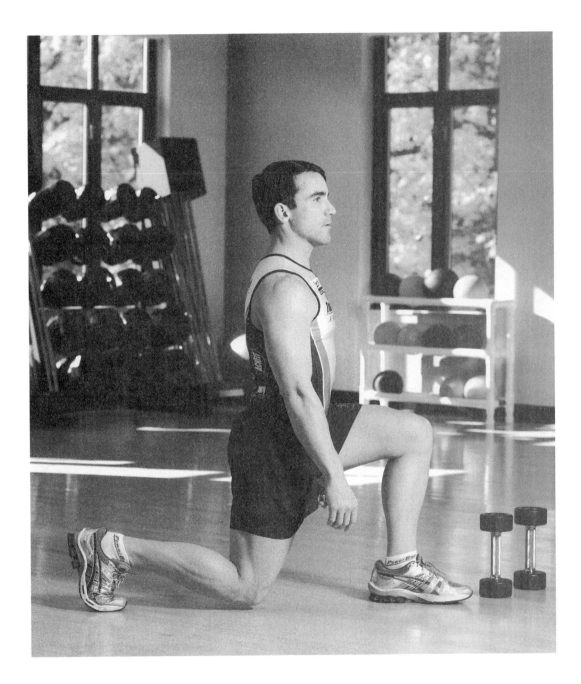

Regular crunch

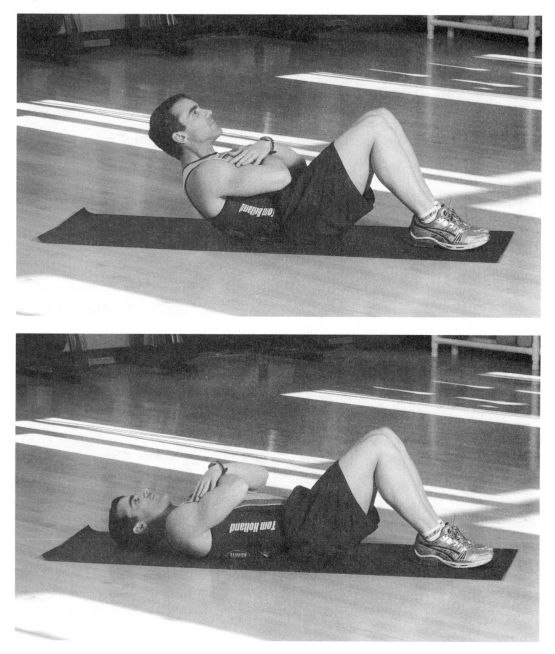

Oblique crunch

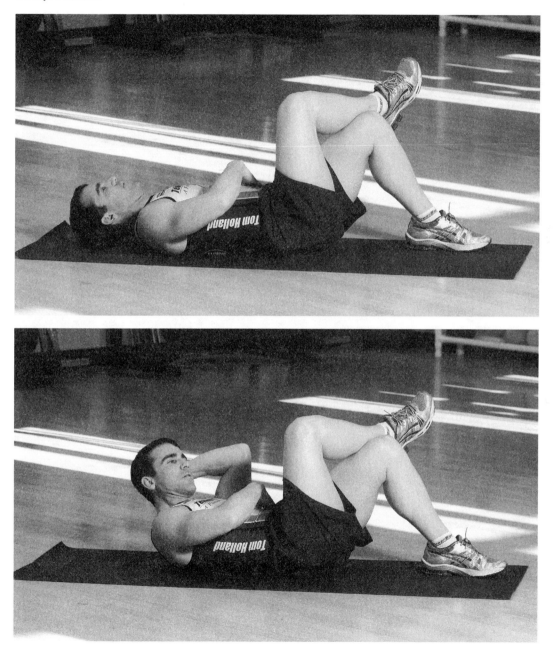

Plank

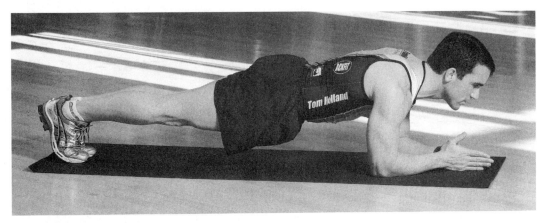

Superman

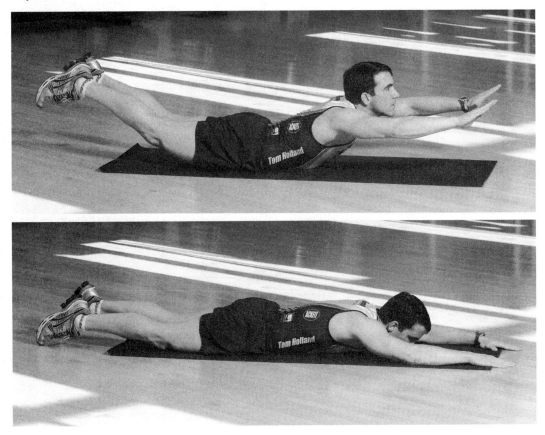

Intermediate Plan A—13 weeks

Exercise	Sets	Reps	Notes
Push up	2	to failure	See Beginner Plan.
Dumbbell row	2	12	See Beginner Plan.
Squat (dumbbells optional)	2	15	See Beginner Plan.
Front lunge (dumbbells optional)	2	15 each leg	Stride forward with one leg until the back knee almost touches the floor, making sure you keep your knees behind your toes and your chest up. Push off and return to starting position. See photos page132.
Backward lunge (dumbbells optional)	2	15 each leg	Stride backward with one leg until the back knee almost touches the floor, making sure you keep your knees behind your toes and your chest up. Push off and return to starting position, then switch legs. See photos page133.
Walking lunges (dumbbells optional)	4	10 steps	Walk across the floor, keeping your knees behind your toes and your chest up.
Calf raise	1	15	Stand with your toes on a step, and hold on to something for support. Drop your heels toward the ground, then raise your body as high in the air as you can by pressing down on your toes. Lower down to starting position. See photos page134.
Core Exercises			
Regular crunch	1	25	See Beginner Plan.
Oblique crunch	1	25 each side	See Beginner Plan.
Bicycle	1	30 seconds	On your back with your hands behind your head, alternate bringing your right elbow to your left knee and your left elbow to your right knee. Keep abdominals tight throughout. See photos page135.
Plank	1	1 minute	See Beginner Plan.
Superman	2	15	See Beginner Plan.

Front Lunge (dumbbells optional)

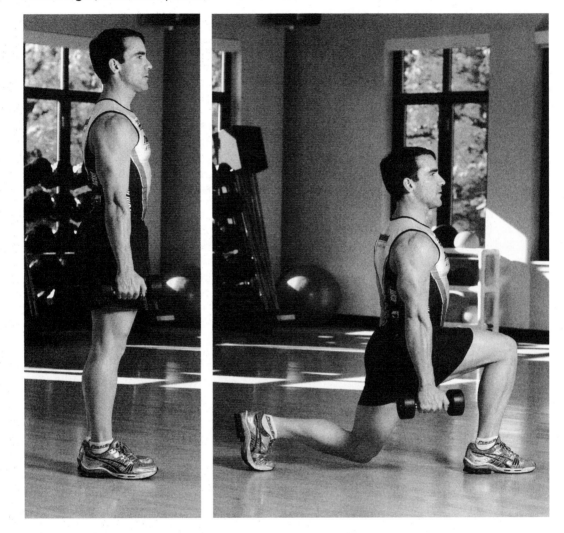

Backward Lunge (dumbbells optional)

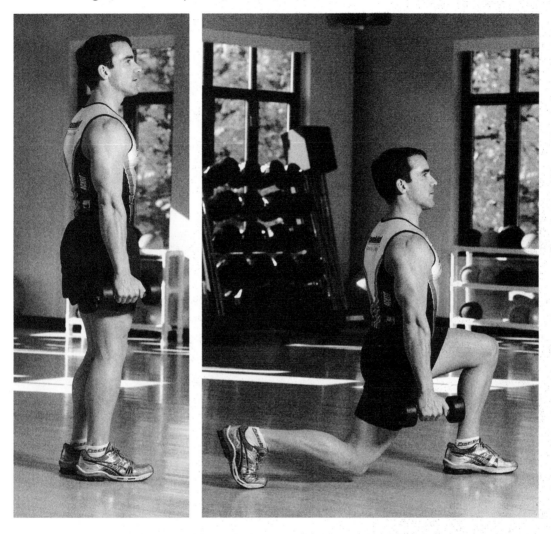

Calf raise

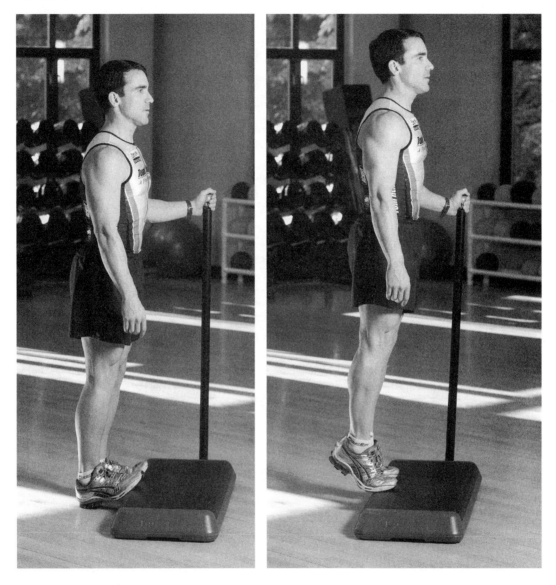

Bicycle

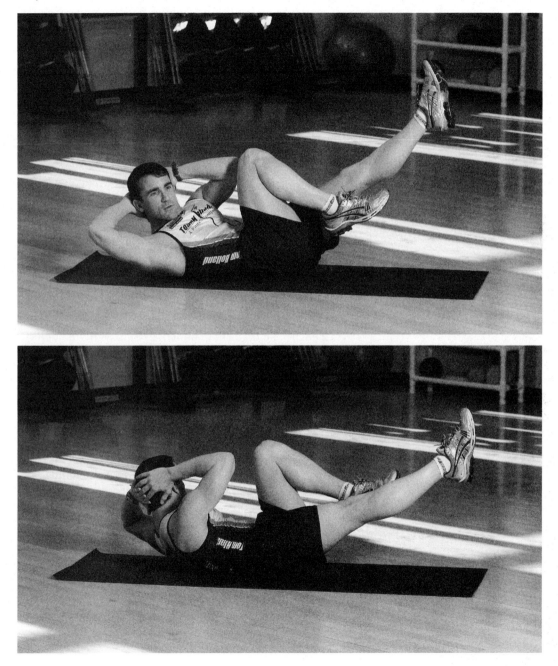

Intermediate Plan B

Base Phase—7 weeks

Exercise	Sets	Reps	Notes
Push up	2	to failure	See Beginner Plan.
Leg extension	2	12	Use leg extension machine. Do both legs together. See photos page 137.
Leg curl	2	12	Use leg curl machine. Do both legs together.
Front lunge (dumbbells optional)	2	15 each leg	See Intermediate Plan A.
Ball squat (dumbbells optional)	2	15	Stand while pressing a stability ball against a wall with your back. Your feet should be a little wider than shoulder-width apart, with your toes pointing forward. Keeping your chest up and knees behind your toes, lower your body down to just above 90 degrees of knee bend, hold for 1 second, and return to starting position. See photos page 138.
Calf raise	1	12	See Intermediate Plan A.
Toe raise	1	12 each foot	Sit on a chair, bench, or ball, with the heel of one foot on a step. Balance a dumbbell or body bar on the toes of one foot. Lift the dumbbell by curling your toes toward your shin, lower down to the ground, and raise back to starting position. See photos page 139.

Core Exercises

Exercise	Sets	Reps	Notes
Back extension	2	10	Use back extension machine. Keep hands pressed to chest, bend at waist, and raise back up until you are perfectly straight, squeezing with your lower back muscles. See photos page 140 and 141.
Oblique crunch	1	25 each side	See Beginner Plan.
Bicycle	1	30 seconds	See Intermediate Plan A.
Plank	1	1 minute	See Beginner Plan.

Leg extension

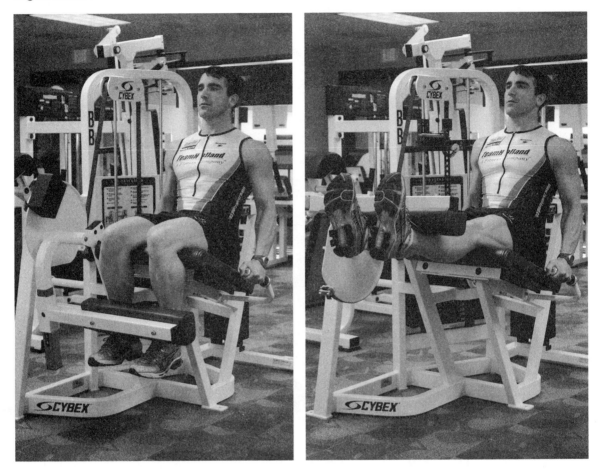

Ball squats (dumbells optional)

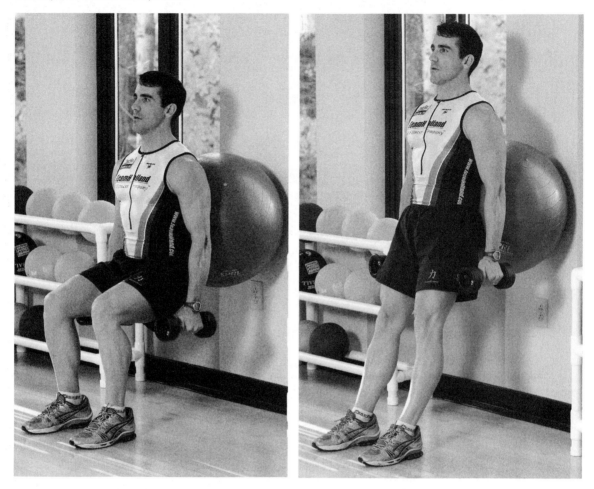

Toe raise

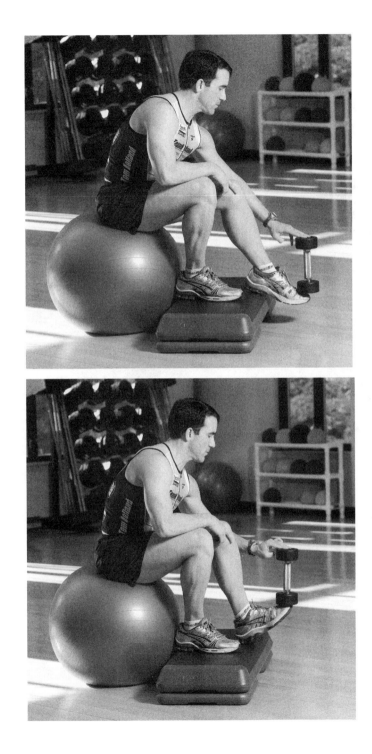

Back extention

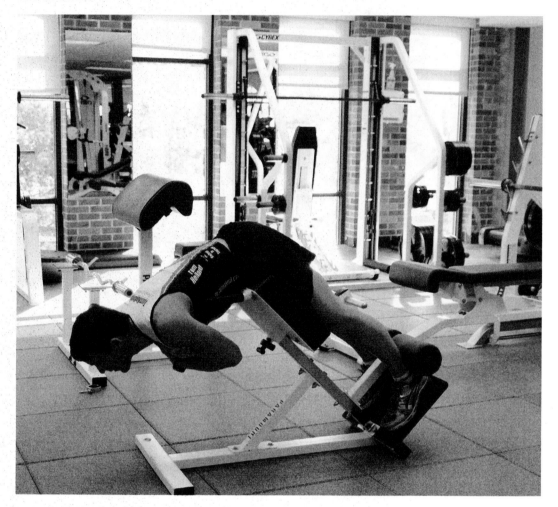

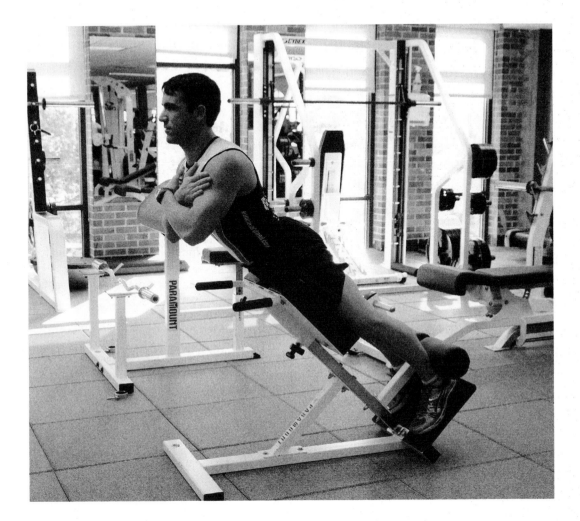

Intermediate Plan B
Build and Peak Phase—6 weeks

Exercise	Sets	Reps	Notes
Push up	2	to failure	See Beginner Plan.
Lat pull-down	2	12	Use a lat machine and grab the bar with a wide grip, with palms facing away from you. Keep shoulders down and pull bar to middle of your chest. See photos pages 143.
Front and back lunge combo (dumbbells optional)	2	10 each leg	Making sure you keep your chest up and your knees behind your toes, step forward with your right leg until your back knee almost touches the floor. Return to starting position without touching the foot to the floor, and then immediately stride backward until that back knee almost touches the floor. Return to starting position and repeat. See photos page 142 and 143.
Step up (dumbbells optional)	2	15 each leg	Place your right foot on a bench no higher than knee height. Step up and tap your left foot on the bench while fully extending your right leg. Step down with left leg and immediately repeat. See photos page 144.
Single leg extension	2	10 each leg	Using the leg extension machine, extend one leg until it is straight, hold for one count, slowly lower it, and then switch legs. See photos pages 147.
Balance board squat	2	15	Standing on an unstable surface, such as a balance board, balance disc, or Bosu, perform regular squats. See photos page 148.
Calf raise	1	12	See Intermediate Plan A
Toe raise	1	12 each foot	See Intermediate Plan B

Core Exercises

Seal	1	15	Similar to the Superman but with your hands at your sides and palms facing up. Lift your chest and feet simultaneously, hold, and lower. See photos page 149.
Oblique crunch	1	25 each side	See Beginner Plan.
Bicycle	1	1 minute	See Intermediate Plan A.
Plank with raised leg	1	1 minute	Perform the plank (see Beginner Plan) while alternately raising and lowering a foot. See photo page 150

Lat pull-down

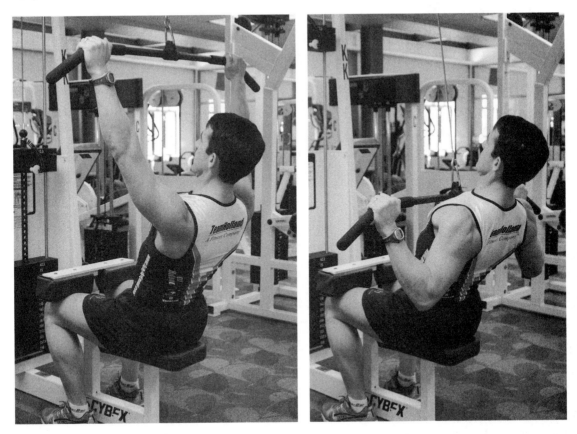

Front and back lunges (dumbells optional)

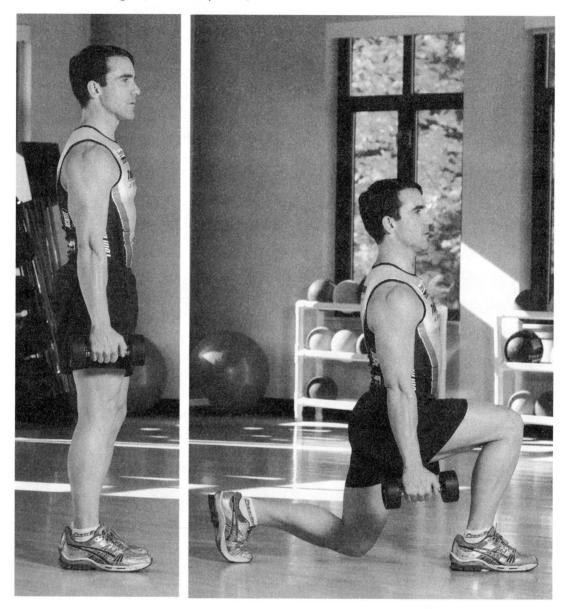

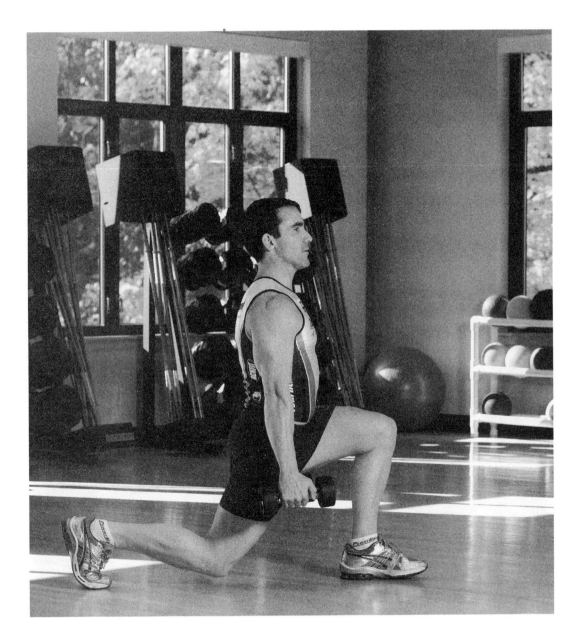

Step up (dumbells optional)

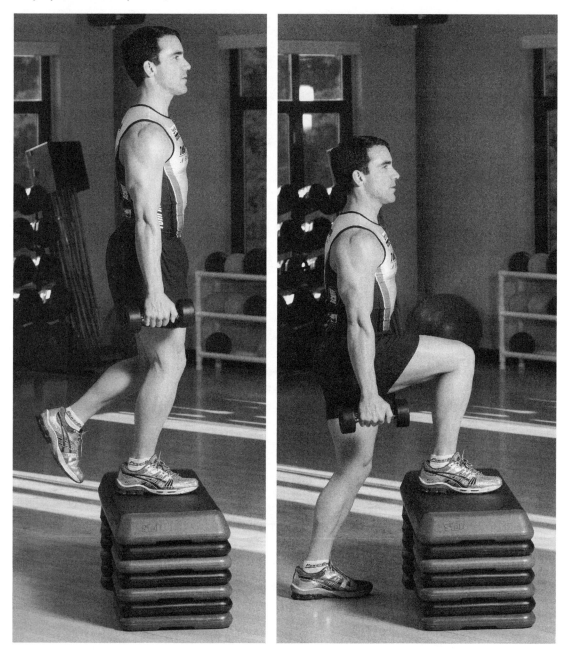

Single leg extension

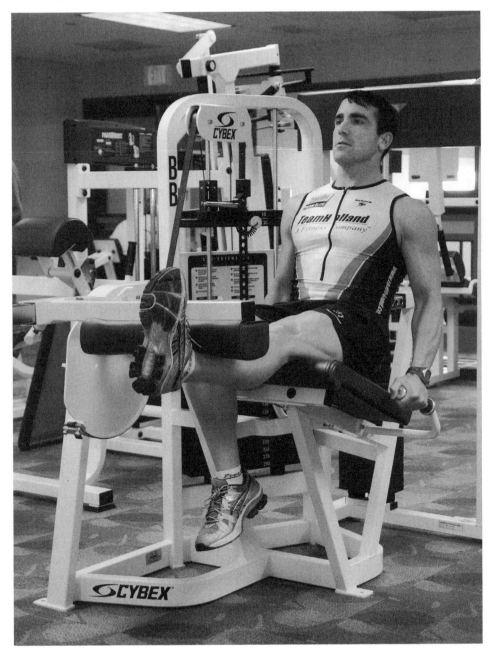

Balance board squat

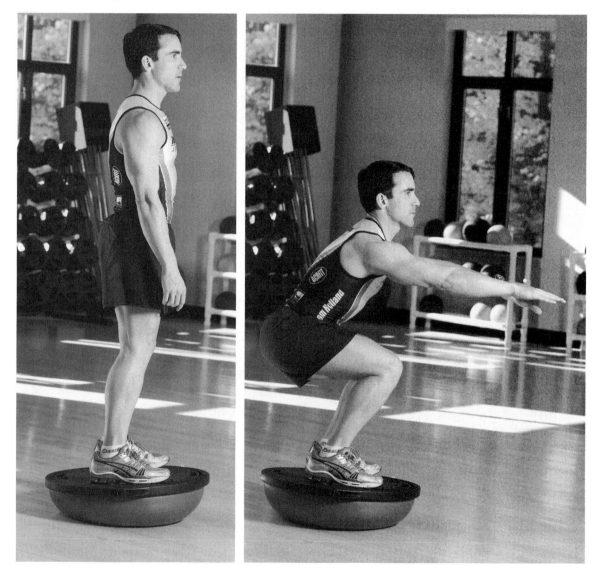

Seal

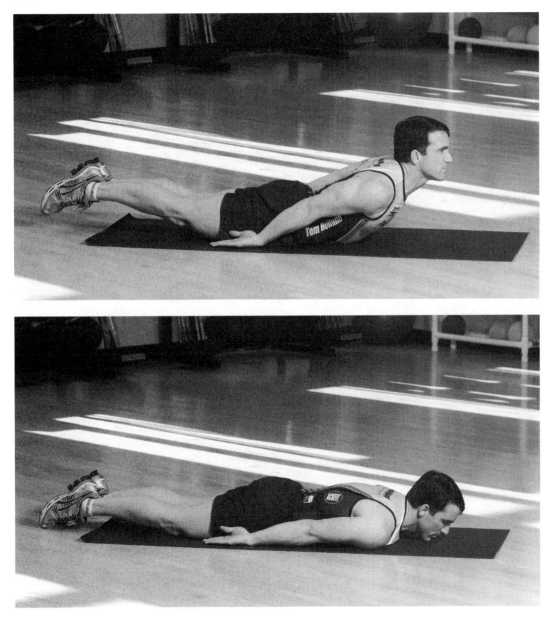

Plank with raised leg

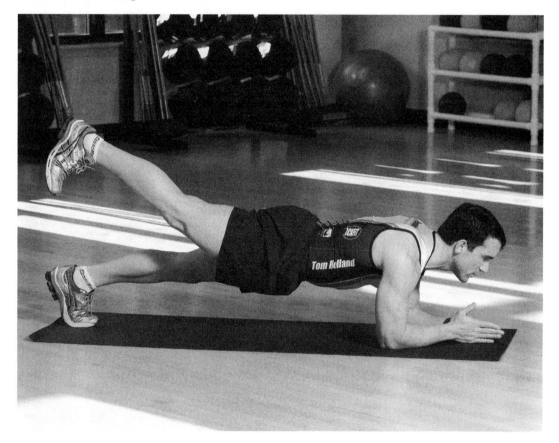

Advanced Plan

Exercise	Sets	Reps	Notes
Barbell squat	2	12	A regular squat (Beginner Plan) but with a barbell resting across your shoulders. See photos page 152 and 153.
Leg press	2	12	Use the leg press machine. Do both legs at the same time. See photos page 154.
Leg extension	2	12	See Intermediate Plan B.
Leg curl	2	12	See Intermediate Plan B.
Calf raise	2	12	See Intermediate Plan A.
Toe raise	2	12	See Intermediate Plan B.
Push up	2	to failure	See Beginner Plan.
Lat pull-down	2	12	See Intermediate Plan B Build and Peak Phase.
Core Exercises			
Regular crunch	2	25	Hands behind your head with legs bent to 90 degrees and raised in the air. Raise your shoulders off the floor while bringing your knees toward your chest. Lower your upper body back down while extending your legs. Repeat. Keep lower back on the floor at all times.
Oblique crunch	2	25 each side	See Beginner Plan.
Reverse crunch	1	20	Raise your head and shoulders off the floor and relax your neck. Extend your arms off the floor at your sides with your palms raised. Raise your legs and bend them to 90 degrees, keeping your lower back on the floor; extend your legs away from you and then back again. See photos page 155.
Superman	1	10	See Beginner Plan.
Bicycle	1	1 minute	See Intermediate Plan A.
Plank	1	1 minute	See Beginner Plan.

Barbell squat

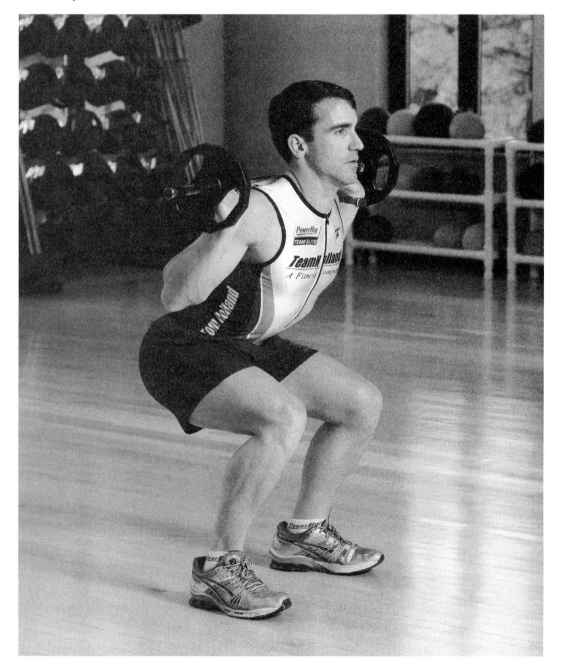

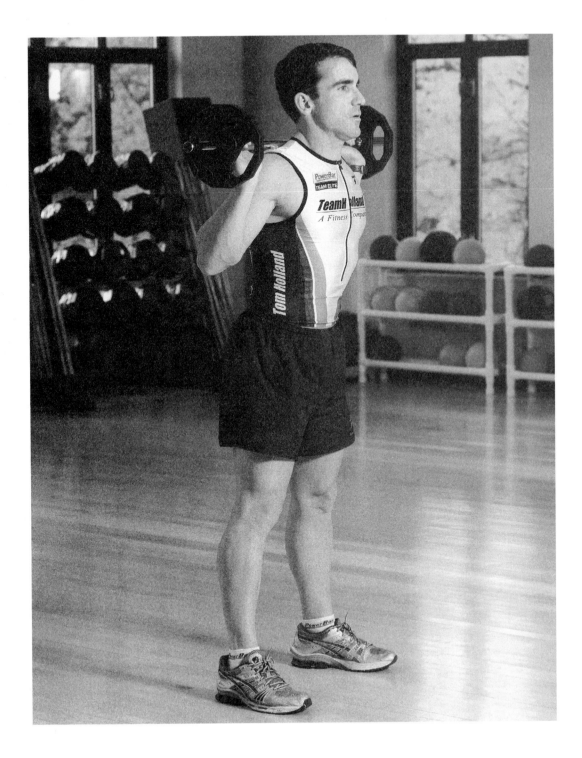

Leg press

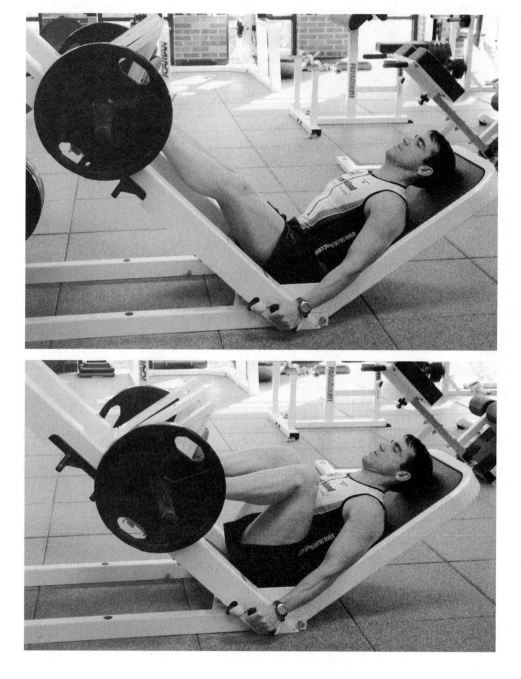

Reversed crunch

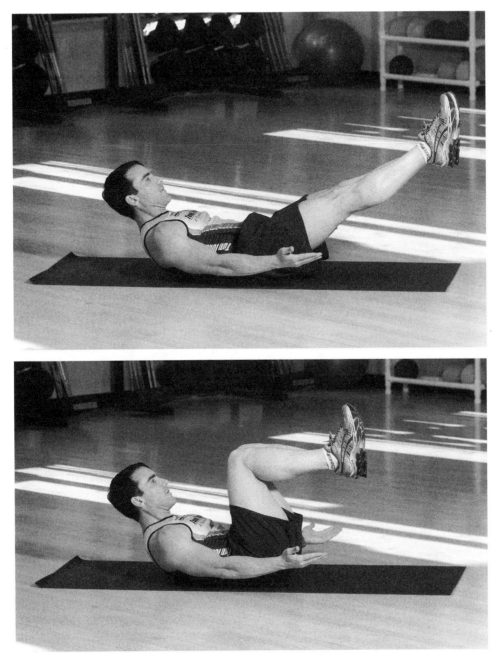

Base #2 and Build Phase—6 weeks

Exercise	Sets	Reps	Notes
Single-leg ball squat (dumbbells optional)	2	10 each leg	Stand on one leg while pressing a stability ball against a wall with your back. Keeping your chest up and knee behind your toes, lower your body to just above 90 degrees of knee bend. Hold for 1 second and return to starting position. See photos pages 158 and 159.
Step up	2	15 each leg	See Intermediate Plan B Build and Peak Phase.
Single-leg dead lift (dumbbells optional)	2	10 each leg	Stand on one leg with knee slightly bent. Keeping your back flat and back leg extended behind you, reach forward and touch the ground with one hand. Return to starting position. Try to balance the entire time. You may add dumbbells as you progress. If you do, you will not touch the ground but pause when you feel the stretch in the back of your leg. Keep your back flat throughout the entire movement. See photos pages 160 and 161.
Balance board squat	2	15	See Intermediate Plan B Build and Peak Phases.
Balance board lunge	2	10	Stand with one leg forward on an unstable surface, such as a balance board or balance disc, and perform stationary lunges. You can also do this with your back leg on a step or bench. See photos pages 162 and 163.
Ball hamstring curl	2	15	Lie with your back on the floor, hips raised, and heels on a stability ball. Pull the ball to your butt and return to starting position. Do not allow your hips to touch the floor throughout the exercise.
Calf raise	1	15 each foot	See Intermediate Plan A.
Cable row	2	12	Use seated cable row machine. Lean forward at the waist with arms extended and lean back while pulling the handle underneath your chest, focusing on pulling with your back muscles. Keep shoulders down and chest out throughout the exercise. If the cable is unavailable, substitute the seated back row machine. See photos pages 164 and 165.

Toe raise	1	15	See Intermediate Plan B.
Box jump*	2	15	Stand in front of a stable box or step no higher than knee height. Jump onto it with both feet and back down again. As you become stronger, you can raise the height of the step and increase the speed of your jumps on and off. See photos pages 166 and 167.

Core Exercises

Ball push up with crunch	3	10	Assume a push-up position with your feet on a stability ball. Do a push up and then pull the ball toward you while keeping your hips high in the air, and then return to starting position. See photos pages 168 and 169.
Plank	1	2 minutes	See Beginner Plan.
Side Plank	1	1 minute each side	Lie on your side with one arm bent underneath you at 90 degrees and your opposite arm resting on your body. Raise your hips and legs off the ground until your body forms a straight line and hold. See photos page 170.
Side-lying obliques	1	20 each side	Lie on your right side with your left arm behind your head, knees bent to 90 degrees, and right arm on the floor in front of you for balance. Bring your elbow toward your hip as you lift your legs off the grond. Lower down and repeat. See photos pages 171.
Back extension	2	15	See Intermediate Plan B.

*High-intensite plyometric exercises. These should only be performed after you have established a significant strength base.

Single-leg ball squat (dumbells optional)

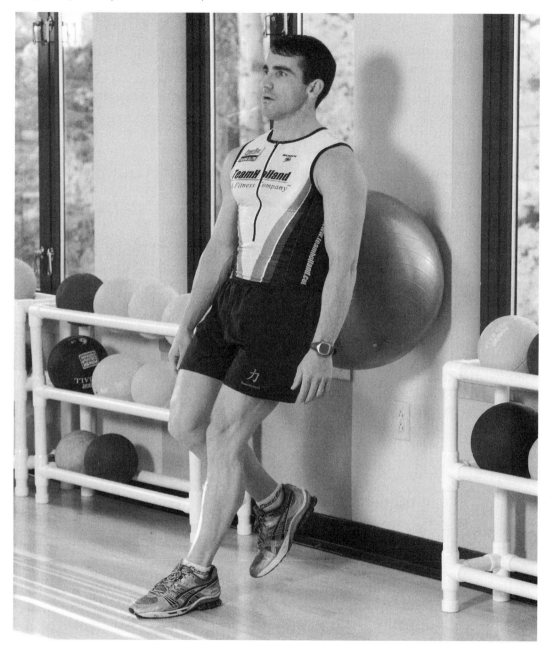

Single-leg ball squat (continued)

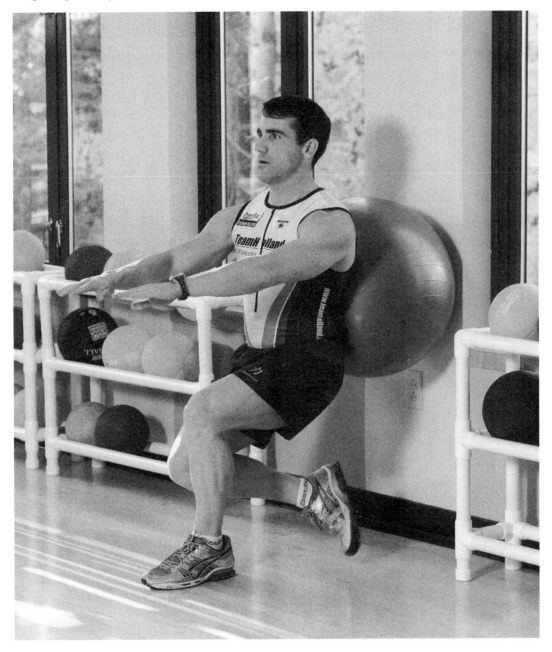

Single-leg dead lift (dumbbells optional)

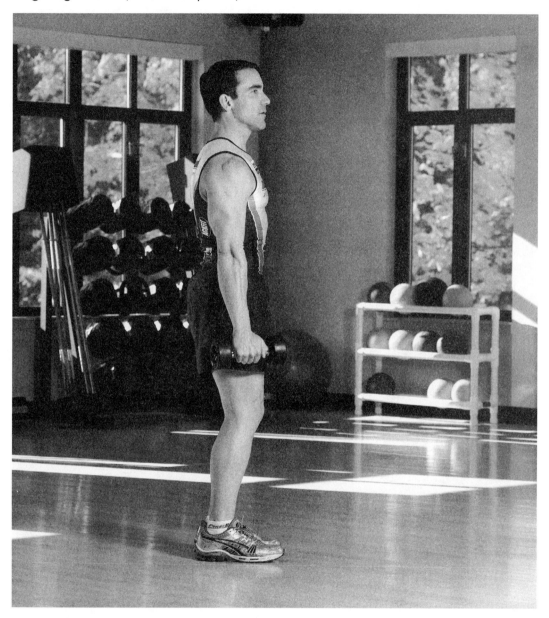

Single-leg dead lift (continued)

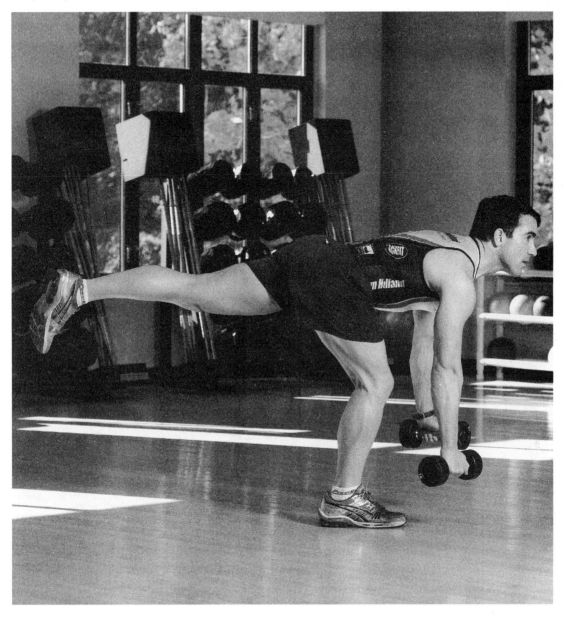

Balance board lunge

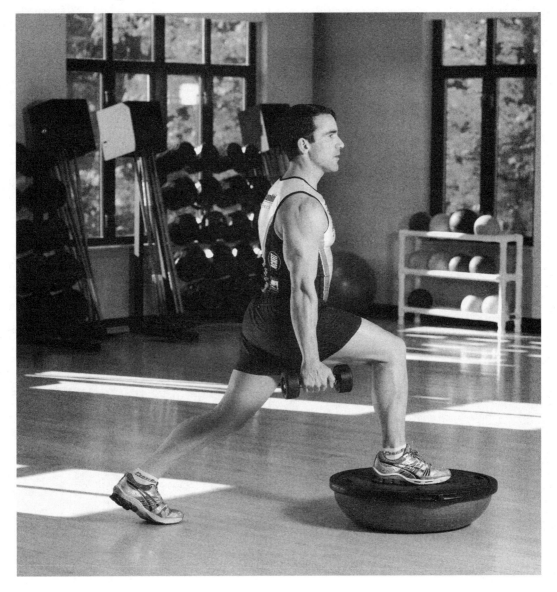

Balance board lunge (continued)

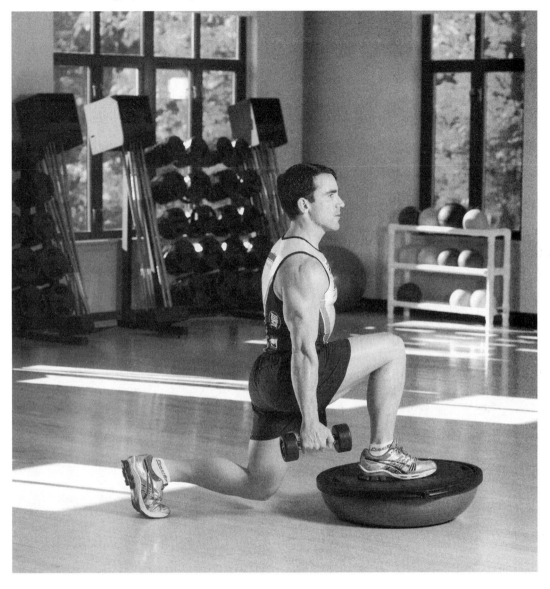

Cable row

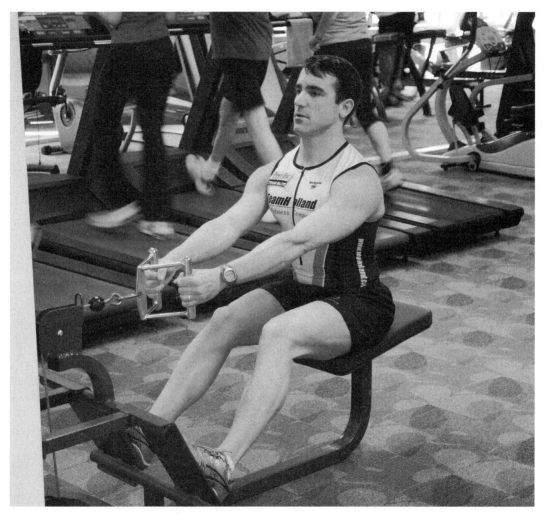

Cable row (continued)

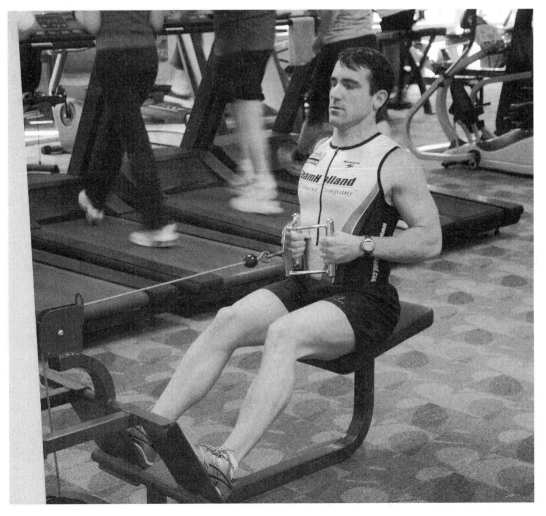

Box jump

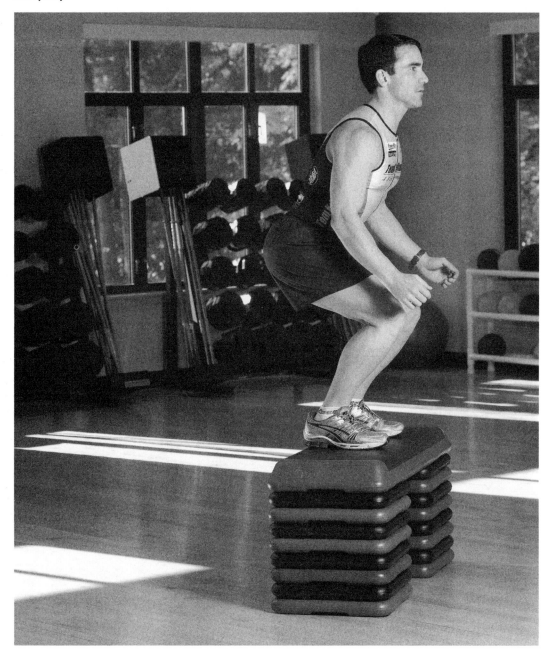

Box jump (continued)

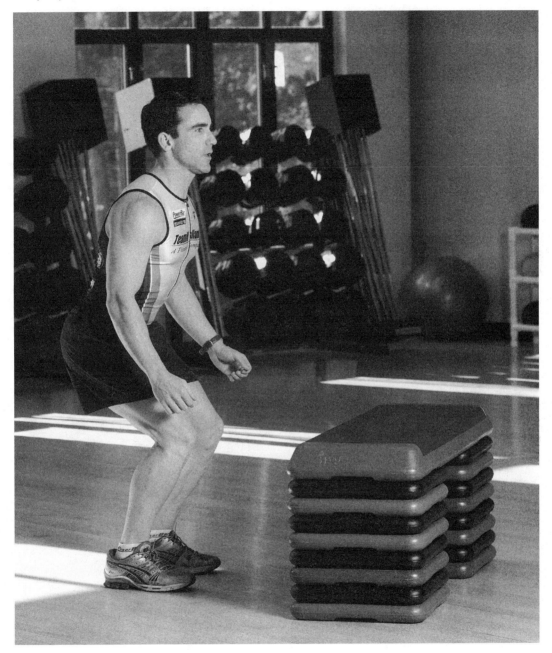

Ball push up with crunch

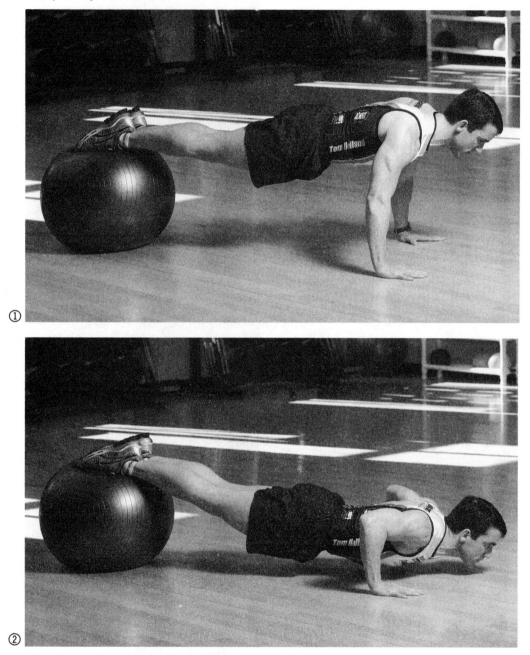

①

②

Ball push up with crunch (continued)

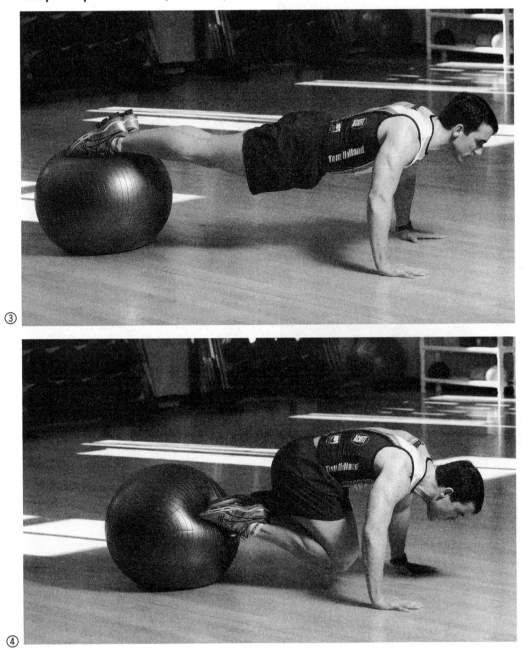

③

④

Side plank

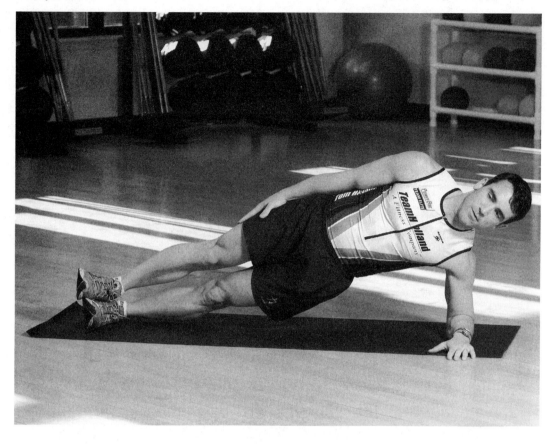

Side-lying obliques

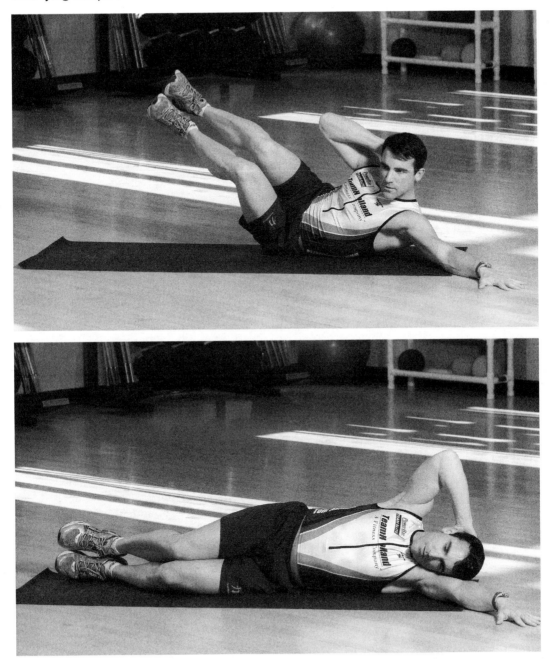

Peak Phase—3 weeks

Exercise	Sets	Reps	Notes
Single-leg ball squat (dumbbells optional)	1	15 each leg	See Base #2 and Build Phase.
Single-leg dead lift (dumbbells optional)	1	15 each leg	See Base #2 and Build Phase.
Balance board squat (dumbbells optional)	1	15	See Intermediate Plan B Build and Peak Phase.
Balance board lunge (dumbbells optional)	1	15 each leg	See Base #2 and Build Phase.
Single-leg ball hamstring curl	1	15 each leg	Similar to the ball hamstring curl (see Base #2 and Build Phase), but using one leg instead of two, pull ball toward you with one leg, and then alternate legs. See photos page 174.
Calf raise	1	15	See Intermediate Plan A.
Toe raise	1	15 each foot	See Intermediate Plan B.
Box jump*	3	15	See Base #2 and Build Phases.
Split box jump*	3	15	Stand on a box or bench no higher than knee height. Jump to the ground with your feet on either side of the box and jump back up. As you become stronger, you can raise the height of the box and increase the speed of your jumps on and off. See photos page 175.
Single-leg box jump*	3	10 each leg	Similar to the box jump (see Base #2 and Build Phase) but using one leg at a time. The box should be much lower, starting just a few inches off the ground. Jump on and off with the same leg for 10 repetitions, then switch legs. As you become stronger, you can raise the height of the box and increase the speed of your jumps on and off. See photos page 176.

Ball wall sit (dumbbells optional)	2	1 minute	Stand while pressing a stability ball against a wall with your back. Your feet should be a little wider than shoulder-width apart, with your toes pointing forward. Keeping your chest up and knees behind your toes, lower your body to just above 90 degrees of knee bend and hold for 1 minute. See photos page 177.
Core Exercises			
Ball push up and single-leg crunch (dumbbells optional)	3	10	The same as the ball push up with crunch (see Base #2 and Build Phase), but this time pulling the ball toward you with one leg, and then alternating legs. See photos page 178 and 179.
Plank with raised legs	1	2 minutes	See Intermediate Plan B Build and Peak Phases.

Single-leg ball hamstring curl

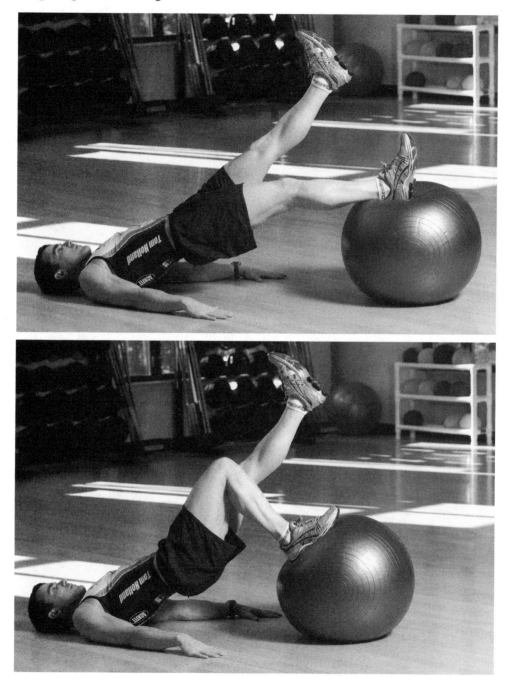

Split box jump

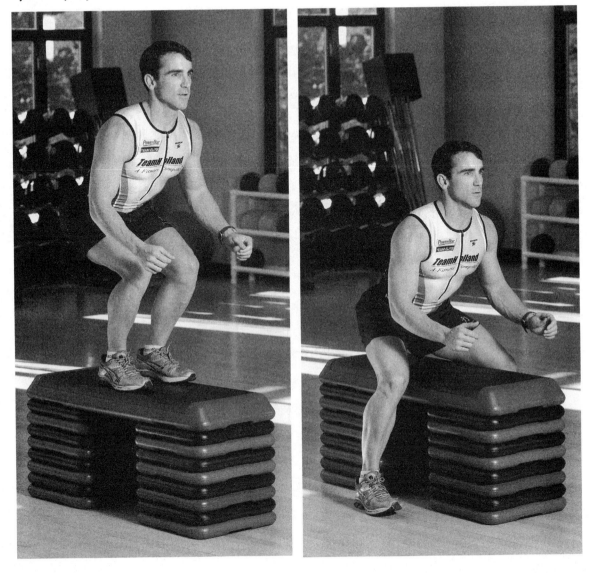

Single-leg box jump

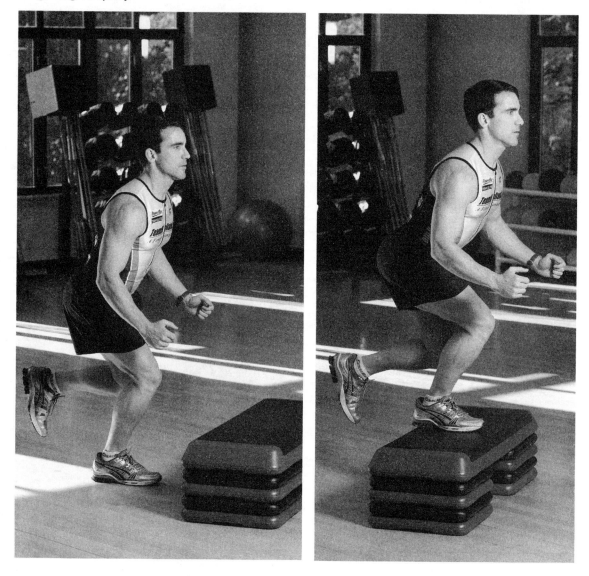

Ball wall sit (dumbbells optional)

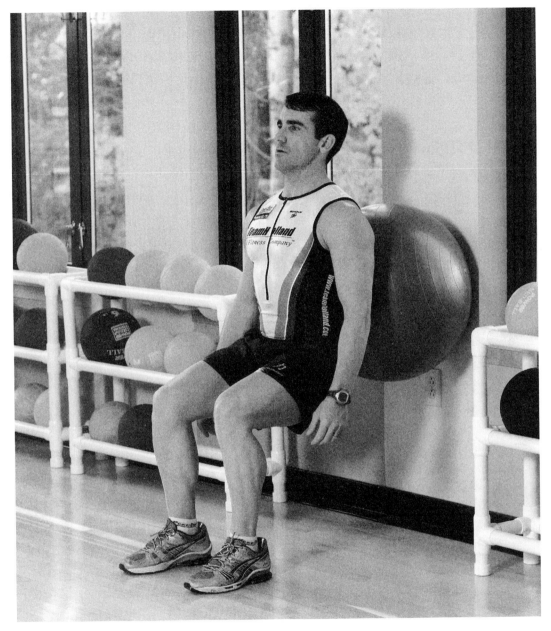

Ball push up and single-leg crunch

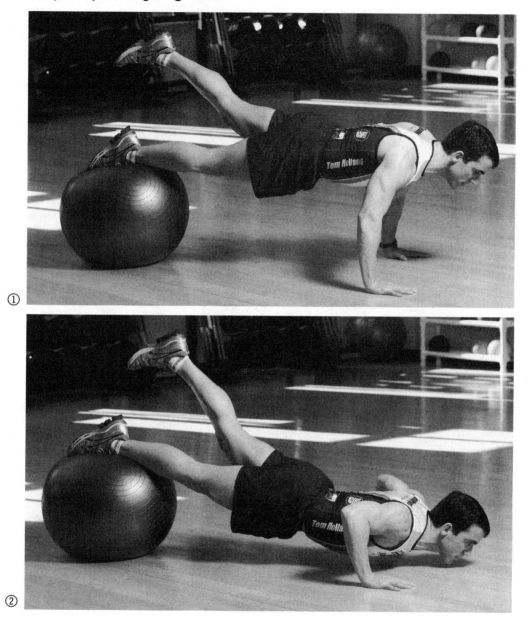

①

②

Ball push up and single-leg crunch (continued)

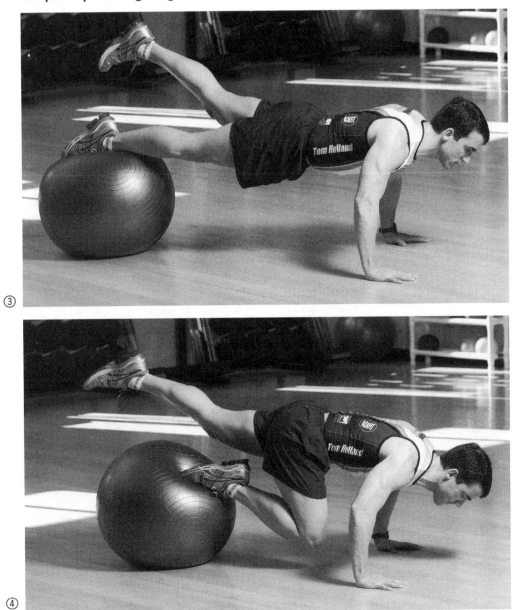

③

④

STRETCHING

If you think there is great debate about the efficacy of strength training for runners, it pales in comparison to the scientific squabbles over stretching. The same arguments apply: Some say that stretching helps runners, while others contend that stretching not only doesn't help, but it also hurts running performance.

Here again, I disagree.

I am not going to launch into a long-winded discussion about the scientific studies that either claim to support or refute the benefits of stretching for runners. Suffice it to say, there are numerous arguments on both sides. Let me just say that the studies against stretching that I have read do not really apply to us as endurance runners. Like the studies concerning strength training and runners, the studies focused on stretching and runners have little applicability to what we do and what our goals are, and their research design is questionable. Much of the research cited on both strength training and stretching for runners has to do with power, not endurance. We are endurance runners. When we run, our muscles get tighter, and when they do, they create imbalances that can lead to injury. It's that simple.

I stretch and my clients stretch. We don't spend a great deal of time doing it, but we do it consistently. I believe that running, especially endurance running, can create tightness in numerous muscles that, if untreated, can cause problems. I find it hard to understand how this point can be argued against, but it is.

Not only is there substantial debate over whether runners should stretch, but there are also differing opinions about what type of stretching protocol to use if you do. There are numerous methods, including ballistic stretching, dynamic stretching, active stretching, passive stretching, static stretching, isometric stretching, and partner assisted stretching.

Here's my philosophy as it relates to stretching:

- Static stretching is the easiest method for alleviating the tightness caused by distance running.

- The optimal time to engage in static stretching is after your run, when your muscles are warm.

- Static stretching involves stretching to the point of tightness and holding for a given amount of time.

- I also employ breathing techniques to increase the effectiveness of the stretch. This involves stretching until I feel tightness, holding, then taking a deep breath in through my nose and exhaling through my mouth. As I exhale through my mouth, I am able to stretch a little further, holding at this new endpoint for a deeper stretch. I repeat this breathing technique several times until I feel I can go no further. I then hold this position for the remainder of the stretch.

- You want to hold each stretch after your run for thirty to sixty seconds.

One of the major roadblocks to stretching is that most runners do not have a set plan for what they are going to do and how long they are going to do it. Runners typically pull up on a toe, push on a tree, and throw in a few lower back twists, and consider that their stretching. There is no structure to the stretching routine.

When you have a distinct progression of stretches, with a set time to hold each one, you are much more likely to do them all. A great benefit to this method is knowing exactly what you need to do and therefore knowing when you are done.

I recommend holding each stretch for thirty seconds. If you are extremely tight and wish to hold them for sixty seconds, be my guest. Use your watch and time each one.

My Super Seven Stretches

The following pages feature the static stretches that I use. The first group is stretches that I perform while standing and the second set is done on the floor. You need to do one stretch per muscle group, but if you want an extra stretch or wish to change your routine a bit, you may add or substitute stretches.

Note: Many runners still perform the hurdler's stretch by stretching one leg in front and bending the other leg into a position that places unnecessary stress on the knee joint. This can be avoided without compromising the effectiveness of the stretch by placing the sole of the bent foot against the inside of the opposite knee.

Do you need to stretch before you run? Marathon runners generally spend the majority of their time running at aerobic paces, at relatively low intensities. When we run at low intensities, the likelihood of pulling a muscle is greatly diminished. The faster we go, the greater the strain we place on our muscles, and the more likely it is that an injury will occur. Thus, for most of our runs as marathoners, stretching beforehand is more of a personal preference than a necessity to improve performance or to prevent injury.

What is indicated or called for before a run workout is known as a "dynamic warm-up." This means that you are in essence "stretching" by means of a low-intensity aerobic activity. For marathon runners, this means that we simply need to start our runs slowly, using the first mile or two as our dynamic warm-up. This gives our muscles a chance to loosen up and our body time to prepare itself for the workout to come.

If you are doing speed work at a track or running a 5K race as a training run, you will need to prepare your muscles a bit more. The significantly faster pace you will be running puts significantly greater stress on the body, and you therefore have a significantly greater chance of pulling a muscle. You still want to begin with a low-intensity dynamic warm-up, such as running at a slow pace for five to twenty minutes. You should then perform some of the static stretches, but you need only hold each one for ten to fifteen seconds.

Seven Stretches and hold each one for thirty seconds, the whole routine will take you just seven minutes.

Stretching can also be a great time to kill two birds with one stone. I like to practice meditation as well as visualization exercises while stretching. This makes the six and a half minutes that much more beneficial.

STANDING STRETCHES

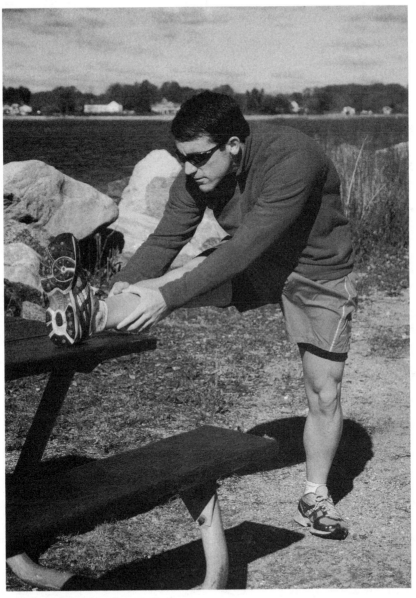

1. Standing Hamstring

Start with a straightened leg up on a stable surface and place your hands on your thigh. Slide your hands down the leg while leaning forward, until you feel a stretch in the back of the raised leg.

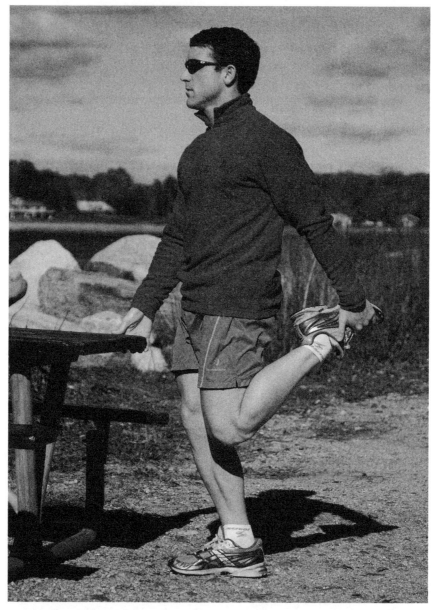

2. Standing Quadricep

Balance yourself with one hand and flex the leg on the opposite side. Keep both knees parallel and gently pull your toes towards your gluteus, feeling the stretch in the front of your thigh. Bend the supporting leg to deepen the stretch; don't swing the bent leg backward.

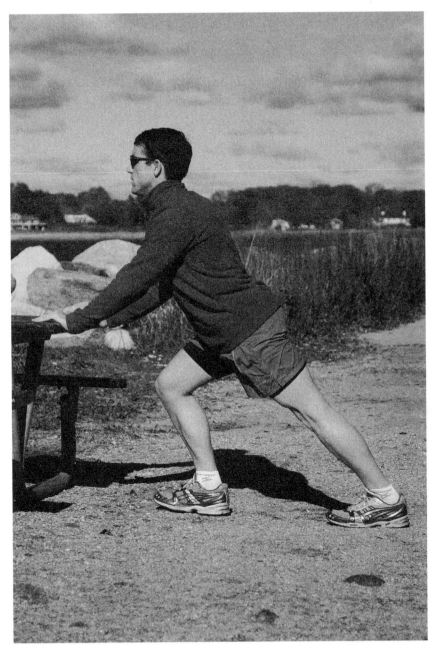

3. Standing Calf

Lean into an object with one leg forward and both heels on the ground. Lean forward slightly until you feel a stretch in the calf muscle in your back leg.

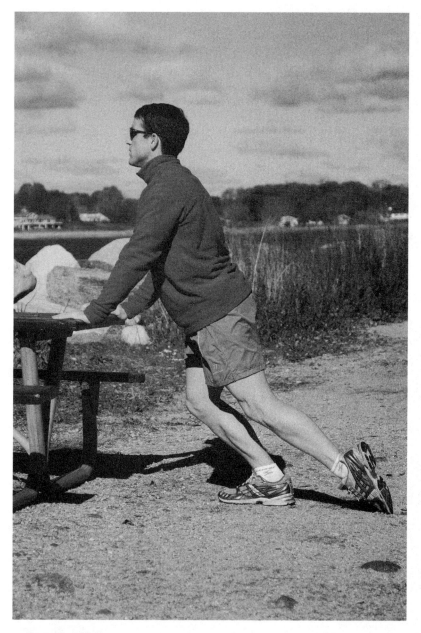

4. Standing Shin

Lean into an object with one leg forward and the top of the toes of your back foot pressed into the ground. Lean forward while pressing the toes into the ground, until you feel a gentle stretch in your shin.

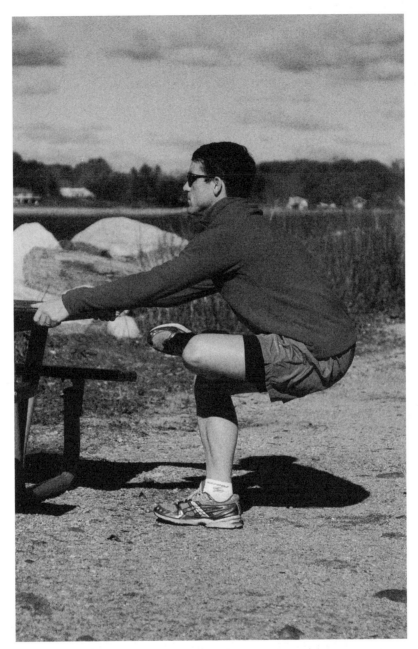

5. Standing Glute

Balance yourself with one ankle crossed over a bent knee. Gently lower your body toward the ground, until you feel a stretch in the gluteus of the raised leg.

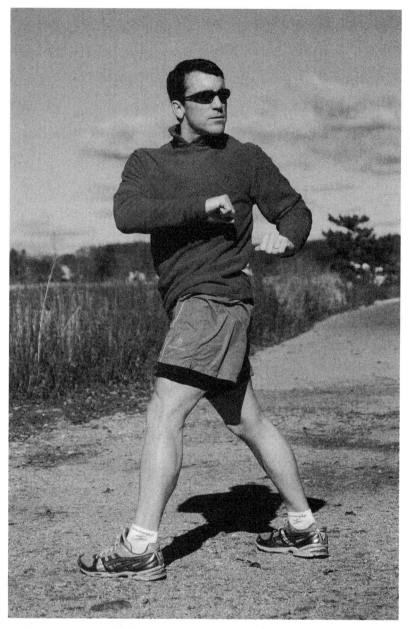

6. Standing Lower Back

Place your hands either on your hips or raise your arms in the air a little wider than shoulder-width apart. Rotate at the hips while twisting your upper body slowly, as far as you can, to the side.

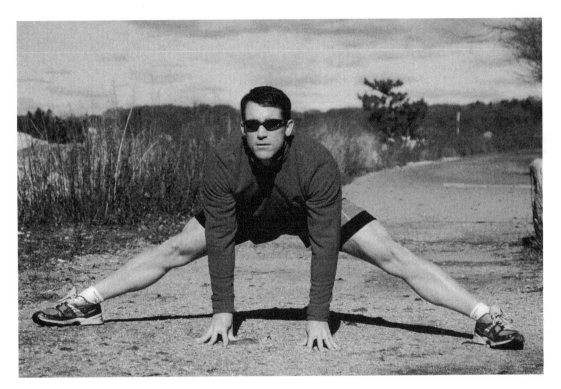

7. Standing Groin

With both feet spread as far apart as possible, slowly lower your upper body and arms toward the ground, until your feel a gentle stretch in the inside of your thighs.

SITTING STRETCHES

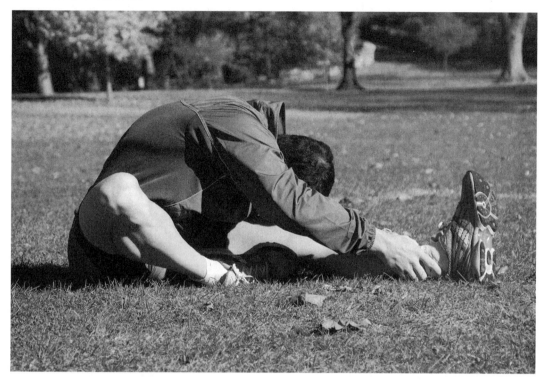

1. Seated Hamstring

Keep one leg straight and the other flexed so that the sole of your sneaker is touching your knee. Bend at the waist while running your hands along the straightened leg toward your foot, until you feel a stretch in the back of your thigh.

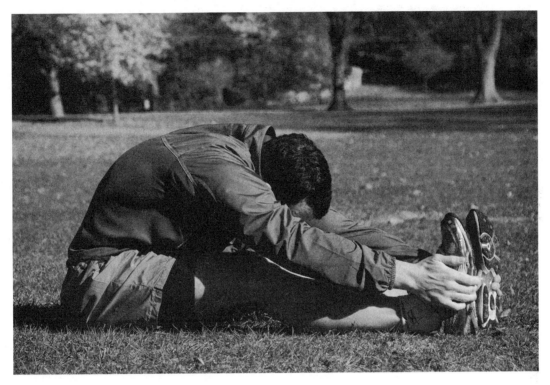

2. Seated Hamstring and Lower Back

Keep both legs straight. While bending at the waist, slide your hands toward your feet, until you feel a gentle stretch in your lower back and behind both thighs.

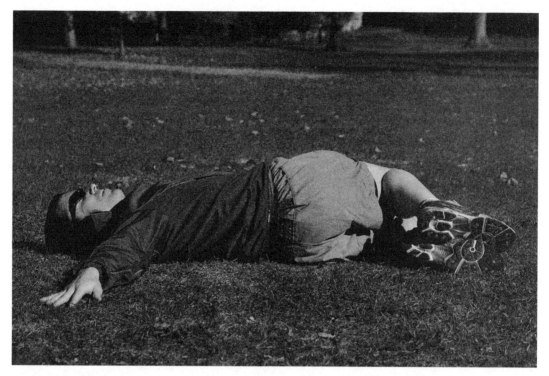

3. Lower Back

Lie with your arms straight out at your sides and your knees raised and bent. Slowly drop both knees to one side, making sure to keep your opposite shoulder pressed against the ground.

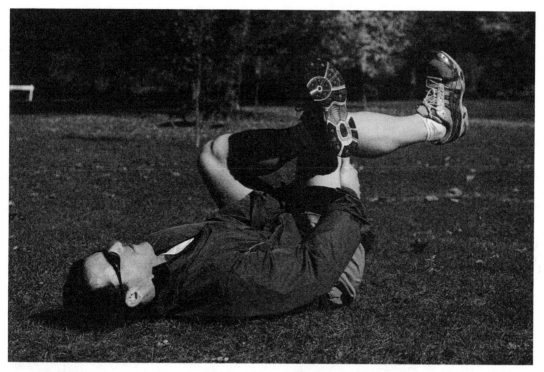

4. Seated Glute

Lie and hold your bent right leg at the thigh with your left ankle crossed in front your right knee. Gently pull your right leg toward your body while feeling a stretch in your left gluteus.

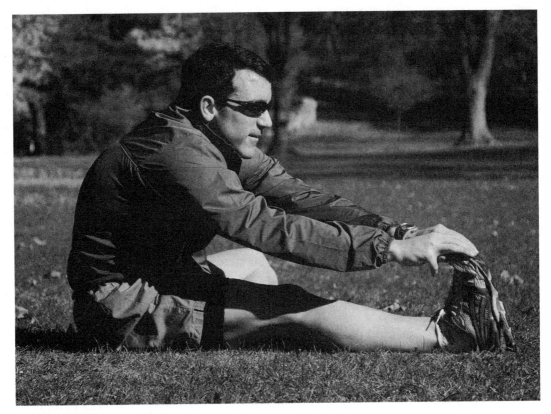

5. Seated Calf

Keep one leg straight and the other flexed so that the sole of your sneaker is touching your knee. Move your hands down the straightened leg, grasp your toes, and pull them toward you while feeling a stretch in the back of your lower leg.

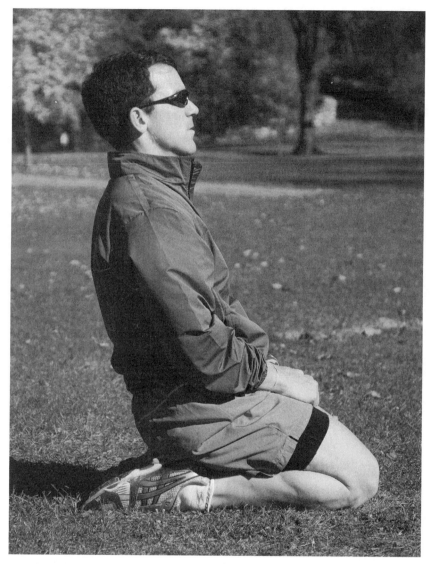

6. Seated Shin

With your feet underneath you and the tops of your sneakers pressing into the ground, slowly lean back slightly while feeling a stretch in the front of your lower legs.

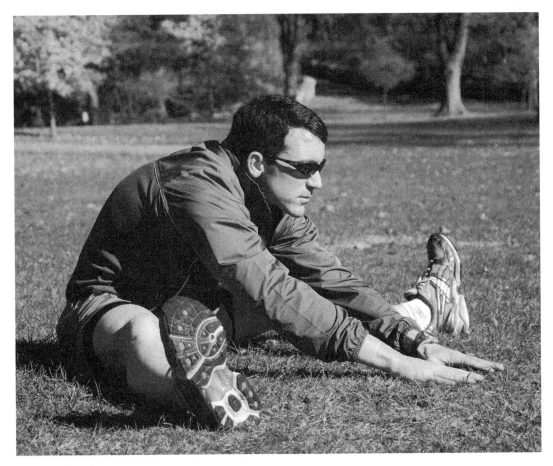

7. Seated Groin

With both legs straight and spread as wide as is comfortable, slowly lean forward at the waist while sliding your hands forward, until you feel a stretch in the inside of your upper thighs.

Running Drills

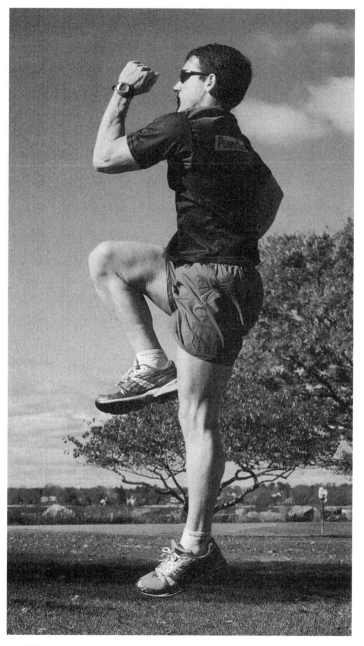

1. Skipping

Move forward and alternate legs. Exaggerate the movements and bound as high as possible while using your arms to propel your body.

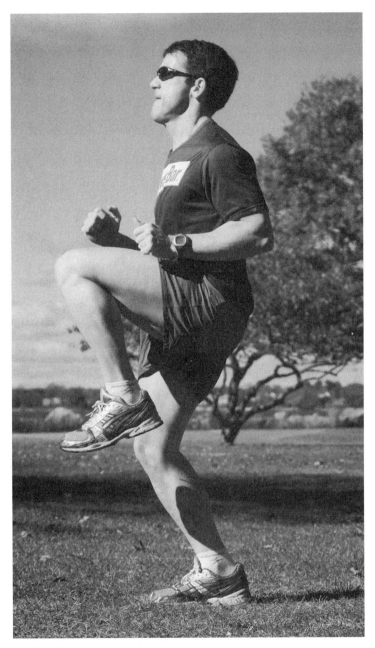

2. High knees

Run forward slowly while pumping your arms. Exaggerate the movements and bring each knee as high into the air and toward your chest as possible.

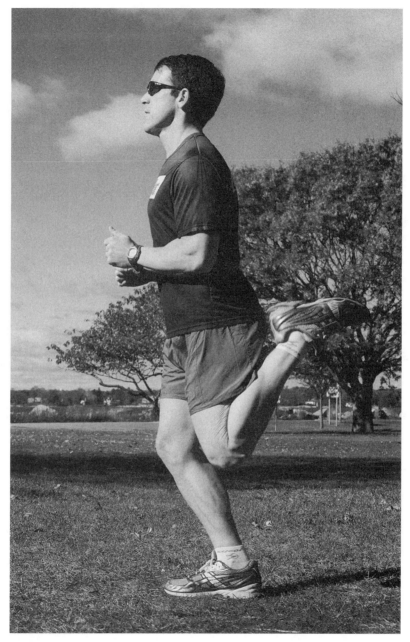

3. Butt kicks

Run forward slowly while kicking yourself lightly in the gluteus with each step.

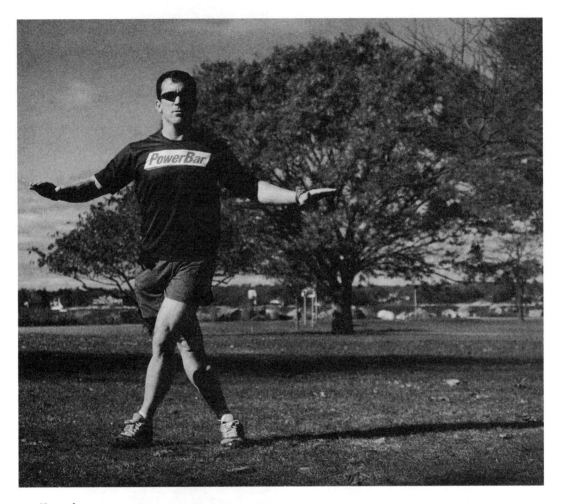

4a. Karaoke

Hold your arms out at your sides and run sideways to the right by alternately crossing your left foot in front of and then behind your right foot. Do the same to the left, using your right foot.

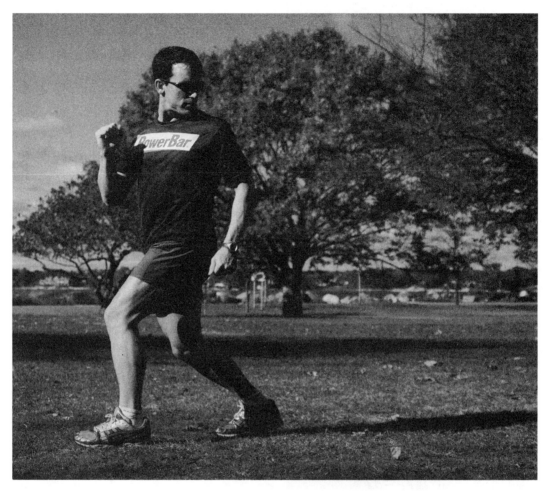

4b. Karaoke

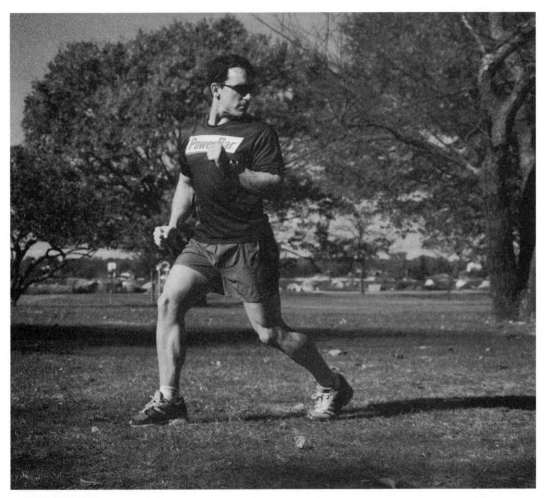

5. Running backward

Lean backward as if you are about to sit in a chair and sprint backward on your toes, pumping your arms and looking over your shoulder as you move.

MY RUNNING DRILLS

You can also perform a few running drills to further warm up the body. (See photos that follow).

You should do each drill one to three times for roughly ten to twenty yards. When possible, try to do them on grass.

I also like to throw in these running drills once a week at the end of a run. They will help your form and flexibility, as well as your body awareness. The entire set of drills takes just five to ten minutes to perform. There is a field behind a school about a quarter mile from my house; at the end of one run per week, I run to this field, do these drills, and then run home.

THE TAPER

I believe a true taper is a major contributor to marathon success. What is a taper? It is simply a gradual reduction in training volume. This allows the body to recover from the weeks upon weeks of training so that you are rested and ready to go come marathon day. Yet, it is much easier said than done. It is extremely hard for people to do, both mentally and physically. You have been training so hard for so long and you become convinced that you will lose fitness if you pull back. Actually, just the opposite is true, but that is a very hard concept for most run-

ners to accept, especially when they are just weeks from their race. It is also very hard to swallow when you see friends and acquaintances continuing to put in major miles in the final weeks before race day. Let them. You are training for an endurance race, not a 100-yard dash. You need to let your body absorb all the hard work that you have been doing. There is a great saying when it comes to overtraining for endurance races:

"It is better to be 10 percent undertrained than 1 percent overtrained."

One of my primary responsibilities as a coach is to ensure that my clients taper correctly. This often includes talking them down and making sure that they adhere to their drastically reduced training schedules when all they want to do is go out and run. When a client calls me during her taper and says that she feels absolutely terrible—she feels fat, sluggish, irritable, and anxious—I reply, "Great!" That tells me that she is tapering perfectly. When you go from running significant mileage to pulling back drastically, as I have you do in the final weeks, your body and your mind will rebel. You will want that running fix, yet you can't have it. You will be burning fewer calories, which can make you feel like you've gained twenty pounds. You will feel slower during the runs you do have left, and this will make you worry even more. Fear not and have faith: You are tapering perfectly. You should spring out of bed on marathon morning and feel like a dog that has been cooped up inside for a week and is raring to go. When in doubt during the final week, leave it out. No one ever ruined a marathon by tapering too hard.

HALF MARATHON

Perhaps you are training to run a half marathon in the hopes that one day you will complete a full one. Or maybe the half marathon is your distance and you have no desire to run 26.2 miles. Whatever the case may be, I have designed several plans for the half marathon as well. I personally love the half-marathon distance: It is just long enough to be challenging yet does not require as much training and overall preparation as a marathon. You can stay in great shape using half marathons as your goal distance.

The half-marathon plans also follow my four-day-a-week running schedule. Almost everything that I have discussed up to this point about preparing for a marathon applies to half marathoners as well. Choose from the same strength-training programs, stretch, do core work, use mental tools, and so on. There are, however, two major differences in preparing for the half rather than the full marathon:

1. You do not really need to carbohydrate-load. Although you certainly want to make sure that you have fuel in your tank by means of carbohydrates, structured carbo-loading is not strictly necessary unless you will be running for three hours or more. You still want to take in fuel during your race, but because you will most likely be running for a relatively short time, you will probably not deplete your glycogen stores.

2. You can run the race a little less conservatively. There is a big difference between running 13.1 miles and 26.2 miles. You can start the half marathon considerably faster than you would a full marathon and push the intensity more throughout the race.

CHAPTER 6
Injuries

As a marathon runner, I am more proud of the fact that I am injury free than I am of my race resume. This is not to say that I am not periodically faced with issues of low-level pain, discomfort, and tight muscles as a result of my running. But I am diligent about addressing these instances immediately, and I set about fixing them before they become a real problem. You can do the same. The glaring conundrum facing runners is that there is a vast number of potential causes of each injury, and it often takes time and a very experienced professional to determine the precise cause as well as the solution. I have found that there are very few people who possess the knowledge to diagnose the etiology of individual running injuries and design an effective course of treatment. Once again, my goal in running is to be proactive rather than reactive and try to prevent pain from arising at all. Lifting weights, stretching, cross-train-ing, following a proper plan, and knowing when to pull back are all essential to injury prevention.

I would recommend that you find a reputable sports doctor in your area. Find a doctor who is an athlete himself or herself, preferably a runner. I would also try to find a sports podiatrist. You need to build a strong network of health professionals who will help keep you fit, injury free, and running for as long as you choose.

Because there are numerous potential causes for the pains associated with running, and many of these causes can create more than one type of injury, having a checklist of these causes can be helpful in self-diagnosing your discomfort. No matter how many qualified doctors you have at your disposal, you will ultimately be the primary caretaker of your body. Through experience and trial and error, you can become very adept at treating these types of issues, making yourself stronger in the process.

POTENTIAL CAUSES OF DISCOMFORT ASSOCIATED WITH RUNNING

1. Running too much too soon

2. Muscular weakness

3. Muscular imbalance

4. Flexibility issue

5. Footwear issue
   - incorrect type of shoe
   - worn-out shoes

6. Running on hard surfaces

7. Running on uneven surfaces

8. Prior injury

9. Too much speed work

10. Not enough rest

11. Biomechanical issue
    - flat feet
    - high arches
    - leg-length discrepancy

When a pain initially presents itself, you can use this checklist to try to identify the possible cause. When a runner tells me that she is experiencing a new running-related pain, my first question tends to be, "What have you been doing differently?" Did she increase her running mileage, change her shoes, or introduce another type of exercise? If a runner has been running for some time and has been pain free, when an issue arises, it stands to reason that something new may be the cause.

Entire books have been devoted to running injuries: their symptoms, treatment, and prevention. In all my years as a coach, there have been a handful of extremely common running-related pains that come up time and again. I will therefore focus on these.

"RUNNER'S KNEE"

Often called "runner's knee," this condition is known formally as chondromalacia patella syndrome or patellofemoral syndrome. People who say they cannot run because of "bad knees" often suffer from this ailment. It is the most common cause of chronic knee pain and is caused by improper tracking of your patella, or kneecap. When the kneecap does not "track" or move correctly, it rubs against bone, causing chronic pain and inflammation. Symptoms include pain during activity such as going up and down stairs, as well as pain associated with sitting with bent knees for extended periods of time. Because the improper tracking of the kneecap is the cause, the goal is to get it into proper alignment. This usually involves strengthening your vastus medialis muscle, the teardrop-shaped muscle on the inside of the front of your thigh. When this is strong, the kneecap will be prevented from tracking to the outside. Leg extensions and isometric quad exercises help strengthen the vastus medialis. Other causes may include prior trauma, improper gait, and increasing mileage too soon. I have found that many people lack the necessary quadriceps strength, and that's why I stress the importance of strengthening the entire lower body through strength training.

When symptoms of chondromalacia patella syndrome present themselves, you should:

1. Decrease mileage.

2. Check shoes for wear and proper fit.

3. Use anti-inflammatories.

4. Apply ice.

5. Cross-train to maintain fitness.

6. Use a **patella strap** for temporary pain management.

Patella strap: This device, essentially a band worn underneath your kneecap, provides compressive support to your patellar tendon and is designed to alleviate symptoms while you run. I am not a proponent of using these indefinitely, because I feel they can become a crutch and keep you from addressing the source of the problem. You can use them, however, as a temporary tool to allow you to continue to run as you decrease your miles and introduce strength training.

It has been my experience that many runners experience chondromalacia patella syndrome at some point in their training, but it is by no means a sign that they cannot or should not run because they have bad knees. What exactly are bad knees? Although I appreciate that some people may have genuine issues that preclude them from running, I believe that most members of this group can run if given the right program. Many people tell me how they tried to run, felt pain, and never tried again. And there are a good number of doctors who tell their patients that running is bad for the joints.

Here's my analogy: Remember when you ate ice cream and had an incredibly painful headache? Did that make you swear off ice cream altogether? Or did you try it again, but this time eating much more cautiously and slowly? The same holds true for the first time you burned your mouth on a scorching hot piece of pizza. Did you never eat pizza again? Of course not. You went back to pizza but approached it in a more mindful way. This may be a gross oversimplification, but I believe it gets the point across: You should apply the same type of logic to running or admit that you simply would rather not run. Or better yet, deal with the problem swiftly and properly, and your so-called bad knees can be cured in a relatively short amount of time without a great deal of interruption to your fitness program.

ICING

Icing your knees when you feel pain will help slow the inflammatory process and lessen your discomfort. When you feel knee pain, such as after a run, you should spend some time icing the affected joints. You can use ice in a plastic bag, a commercially made ice pack, or a bag of frozen vegetables (my favorite method). Ice your knees for five to ten minutes, remove the ice for the same amount of time, and repeat several times through. If I am training especially hard, I will often ice proactively after a workout, even if I am not experiencing pain.

ILIOTIBIAL BAND SYNDROME

The iliotibial band is connective tissue that runs from your hip down to your knee on the outside of your thigh, and it helps stabilize your knee. Iliotibial band syndrome (ITBS) is a friction injury that can cause pain in the hip or on the outside of the knee. This band normally rubs on the outside of the knee, and ITBS is the most common source of lateral knee pain in runners. Causes can include hip abductor weakness, a tight IT band,

overpronation, hard downhill running, running on the same side of the road, and excessive speed work. Once again, by strengthening your lower body, you can help avoid a problem such as ITBS. Hip abductor exercises, such as lying on your side and raising your top leg toward the ceiling, will help strengthen your abductors, as will the seated leg abduction machines at the gym. If the pain is on the outside of the knee, you can treat with ice and anti-inflammatories. Exercises targeting the abductors along with massage can also help alleviate the symptoms. Although there are certain stretches meant to target the IT band, I have found them to be relatively ineffective. But I have found massage to be highly beneficial, both self-massage and by a trained therapist. There are two pieces of equipment that I also recommend to help loosen a tight IT band: foam rollers and a device known as "The Stick."

FOAM ROLLERS

These basic foam cylinders are becoming more and more popular and come in a wide variety of lengths and colors. They really help you work your IT band deeply as you utilize your own body weight to lend pressure. Place the foam roller on the ground and lie on top of it, with the roller positioned underneath your hip. Then roll up and down on top of it, moving the roller from your hip down to your knee and back again. By supporting your body weight with your arms, you can control the amount of pressure and the depth of the massage. When you have a tight IT band, you will feel just how tight it is when you work it on a roller. You should see some improvement after several daily sessions of just a few minutes each.

THE STICK

You hold each end of this simple plastic stick while running it up and down the outside of your thigh from your hip to your knee. Performing this massage-like exercise for a minute or two several times a day can really help loosen a tight IT band.

> **Note:** These pieces of equipment can often be difficult to find in stores. The website www.performbetter.com offers these and many other helpful training tools for runners.

PLANTAR FASCIITIS

The plantar fascia is a band of connective tissue that runs from your heel to the base of your toes. Plantar fasciitis is inflammation of that tissue. A major telltale sign of plantar fasciitis is pain in the bottom of your foot when you step out of bed in the morning. The pain may subside with activity yet resurface after you stop. This condition can worsen if left untreated and you should deal with it immediately once symptoms present themselves. It can be caused by conditions such as high arches, flat feet, running in old sneakers, and tight calf muscles. If you experience this type of early morning foot pain, you should immediately:

1. *Apply Ice.* Freeze a water bottle and roll it back and forth on the ground under your bare foot. Do this for several minutes, take a few minutes off to let your foot warm up, and then repeat several more times through.

2. *Check Your Shoes to Ensure That They Are Not Too Worn Out.* Although many running experts claim that old shoes are not a potential cause of plantar fasciitis, I disagree. I have experienced the symptoms several times, always after I wore running shoes far past the recommended mileage.

3. *Stretch Your Calves.* Tight calves can be a factor in plantar fascia pain. You should perform the calf stretches described in the last chapter, doing them several times a day to loosen your calf muscles. You can also purchase the Step Stretch to add another dimension to your stretching routine and help keep your plantar fascia from becoming tight and inflamed.

4. *Take Anti-Inflammatories.*

If pain persists, you should consult a qualified sports podiatrist. You may be a candidate for custom **orthotics** to correct any biomechanical issues that may be causing your plantar fasciitis, and a sports podiatrist can rule out any other possible causes. Pulling back on your running miles and cross-training is always a good idea until the symptoms subside.

> **Orthotics:** Orthopedic devices designed to treat or adjust various disorders of the foot.

BACK PAIN

Almost everyone experiences back pain at some point in their lives, and the potential causes are almost infinite. Several prominent doctors even believe that many back problems have psychological causes rather than physical. As a runner, my experience has been that back pain is often caused by the following:

1. *Tight Hamstrings:* When the hamstrings are tight, back pain can frequently result. Work in a few extra hamstring stretches throughout the day to help alleviate this possible cause.

2. *A Weak Core:* If your abdominals or your back muscles (spinal erectors) are weak, this can lead to postural problems and ultimately back pain. This is why my strength-training programs contain exercises for both sides of your midsection. Especially during longer runs, if your core is weak, your posture will be compromised, your form will break down, and you might experience back problems.

3. *Tight Back Muscles:* This might be common sense, but unfortunately it is also an all-too-common problem, especially in this day and age when people spend hours upon hours seated hunched over in front of a computer. Performing simple back stretches throughout the day can really make a huge difference. I personally love the back stretch where you lie on your back, bend your knees, and slowly lower them to one side of your body and then the other.

4. *Shin Splints:* As I said earlier, I spent my entire high school football career injured and benched while I nursed excruciating shin splints. Shin splints are pain in the front of the lower leg, or shin area. Although there are several other lower leg conditions with similar symptoms, including compartment syndrome and stress fractures, it has been my experience that shin splints

are much more common. Shin splints are caused by an overload on your shinbone (tibia) and the connective tissue. Shin splints are commonly caused by doing too much too soon, which is what I believe caused my pain during high school. After doing nothing all summer, we then took part in football's "Hell Week," running from dawn until dusk for two weeks straight. Needless to say, many of us became injured as a result.

Too much mileage too soon and too much high-intensity running often cause shin splints. Weak shin and calf muscles, overpronation, and flat feet may also be potential causes. Weak musculature is one reason I include tibia raises and calf raises in the strength-training program.

The exercises involving balance also help prevent this type of injury by increasing the strength and stability of your lower legs. As with all exercise, if you begin to experience this type of pain, you should pull back in your training, use ice and anti-inflammatories, begin targeted strength training, stretch the affected area and opposing muscles as well (calves), cross-train, make sure you are wearing the appropriate footwear, and go over

your training plan to see whether changes need to be made. Thanks to slowly building a solid running base and faithfully doing my lower leg exercises, my shin splints are a distant memory.

5. *Piriformis Syndrome:* The piriformis is a muscle located deep in your glutes. A classic symptom of piriformis syndrome is literally a "pain in the butt," which often presents when you are seated for extended periods of time, such as driving long distances in a car, and it may also become worse with exercise. The pain can also travel down your leg, usually stopping at the knee. A dull ache down in the ankle can also be a symptom.

The piriformis muscle is located near the sciatic nerve, and for some people, it actually runs through this nerve. Thus, when the piriformis muscle irritates the sciatic nerve, pain radiates down through the leg.

If you are afflicted with this syndrome, I recommend that you repeatedly stretch the glutes while manipulating your leg to focus on the piriformis muscle. I also believe that weak abductors may play a large role in piriformis syndrome because the piriformis is forced to absorb more of the intensity involved in running and becomes irritated over time. I have found great success dealing with this syndrome through unilateral weight training to strengthen the abductors and glute muscles of the affected leg. In addition, having a massage therapist work the affected area can be painful but will help stretch the shortened piriformis muscle.

Note: If there is one pain associated with running that I have had a great deal of experience with, it's piriformis syndrome. I began experiencing this pain in 2000, and it plagued me for quite some time. I had endless massages and electric muscle stimulation sessions, and it convinced me to seek the services of a chiropractor. All of the advice I received at the time was reactive rather than proactive. Piriformis syndrome and its causes are a source of debate among sports doctors, and there are some who believe that it doesn't even exist. All I know is that I suffered major pain, and stretching, though it felt good, didn't make it go away. I began to focus on strengthening my hip abductors and glutes in an effort to combat this condition and, lo and behold, the symptoms that I had endured for years disappeared and my running improved dramatically. I believe that all of these exercises, including the advanced one-legged ball squat (see photo page 158) to strengthen my glutes, had a direct impact on curing my piriformis issues.

Remember, running is not bad for your joints and injuries are not unavoidable. Running exposes our individual weaknesses and, if we wish to continue running, forces us to strengthen these weak links. Running, therefore, can truly help us become the best that we can possibly be.

CHAPTER 7
Pre-Race Preparations

You are in the final days leading up to your race. You are tapering correctly, so you are probably going out of your mind. This is a good thing and to be expected. This is also a great time to pull out your training journal and read each entry. It can help increase your confidence exponentially as you recall all the miles you put in that you have long since forgotten.

Make sure that you have everything you need: shoes, race wear, nutrition products, race gear, everything. The last thing you want to do is sprint around the day before the race (or worse yet, the day of) to find that one thing you absolutely, positively must have for the marathon. Plan on having everything you need by Thursday if your race is on Sunday; this will afford you a small buffer zone if you run into problems. Do not take this advice lightly; you want the final days before your marathon to be as stress-free and relaxing as possible.

MARATHON STRESS DREAM

There is an interesting phenomenon that affects almost all marathoners at some point in their training. It's what I like to call the Marathon Stress Dream. It can strike at any time, but the first one typically shows up a couple of months before your race. You are thinking about your marathon more and more as the weeks pass, and much of this gets pushed down into your subconscious. Inevitably, you will have a dream (or should I say nightmare?) about your marathon, in which something or everything goes wrong. You may have a Seinfeldian dream where your alarm clock does not go off and you oversleep. Or you realize as you are running that you have forgotten to put your chip on your shoe. Maybe you dream that you take a wrong turn and end up lost, or perhaps you combine an old familiar nightmare with the stress of the marathon and dream that you are running the marathon completely naked. These dreams can become increasingly bizarre and even humorous, and there is an amazing sense of relief when you wake from one to realize that it has all been in your mind. Just know that this is very common. I still have them, and I'm sure the top professional runners experience them as well.

PUTTING YOUR NAME ON YOUR RACE SHIRT

Many runners like to write or have their names printed on the shirt they intend to wear during their marathon. Some write their names on with magic marker; others like to have their names printed professionally. If you opt for the professional method, do not wait until the last minute to have it done. Having your name on your shirt allows spectators to cheer you on, which can help immeasurably, especially when the going gets tough. I highly recommend this practice, especially for first-time runners. If you plan on doing this, remember to wear the same shirt while training, not just on race day. Also, be sure to put your name on a shirt that will be appropriate for the expected temperature, and be prepared to change if the conditions warrant. Putting your name on a long-sleeve shirt and having the temperature rise into the high seventies or eighties can prove disastrous. You may want to put your name on several different shirts and on race morning choose the one that corresponds to the current temperature. Or you can just write your name on your shirt or arm with a magic marker on race morning.

KNOWING THE COURSE

In my experience, runners can be divided into two groups: those who want to know every detail about the course beforehand and those who want to see it for the first time on race day. Both approaches are fine; you need to do what will make you the most comfortable. I have clients who insist on driving the entire course before the race and others who would rather see it on foot. I do, however, urge you to learn as much about the race as you can so that you experience no surprises. Some races even provide guided tours of the course. You may receive information in the mail and/or by email; I also encourage you to visit the race website (if there is one) and review it thoroughly. Print out any documents that you might need to have with you. Make sure you know where you need to be, at what time, and how you will get there. The start line for some races is very easy to get to, while others can only be reached in very specific ways, which is the case with the New York and Boston marathons. The more you know about the race, the less stressed you will be.

DESTINATION MARATHONS

If you are traveling some distance to your marathon, especially by plane, you must make sure that you have everything you need before you leave. Do not assume that you can purchase an essential item or items after you arrive. Running a marathon in Rome? Maybe you won't be able to find that orange Gatorade you need, or any Gatorade, for that matter. If you absolutely must have a certain type of oatmeal for breakfast, be sure to pack it. Bring everything with you that you possibly can. As I stated earlier, I often ship my special drinks and other gear to my destination ahead of time. Doing this frees me from having to drag these things along as I travel, especially something as heavy as drinks in plastic bottles, which can also burst in transit. Furthermore, in this era of ever-tightening airport security, anything you can ship ahead of time is one less potential headache or, worse yet, confiscated item. I have had armfuls of necessary race items confiscated from me while en route to races. Air travel presents a dilemma with your essential race gear; putting it in your checked luggage can help avoid confiscation and hassles at security, but when you check luggage, your gear might get lost or damaged. I recommend wearing your race sneakers or packing them in your carry-on bag, along with any items that you must have and that you cannot afford to be without should your luggage get lost. Spending a few extra dollars to ship items ahead of time can often make traveling much easier both mentally and physically.

Top Two Marathons with Fastest Median Times

	1995	2000	2004
Philadelphia	3:41:47	4:01:19	4:04:38
Cleveland	3:55:51	3:57:04	4:05:47

Source: www.marathonguide.com

MY HONOLULU MARATHON EXPERIENCE

In 2006 my in-laws invited my wife and me to vacation with them on the Big Island of Hawaii. Running junkie that I am, I jumped on the Internet to see whether there would be any races during our stay. Sure enough, the Honolulu Marathon was taking place right when we would be passing through on our way to Kona. I arranged our itinerary so that I would be able to run the marathon; we would stay overnight in Honolulu, I would race the next day, and we would fly out that night.

As we would only be in Honolulu for a short time, our schedule was very tight and would not allow for much flexibility. We made it to the expo to pick up my race packet and number just before it closed, and then went to our hotel, which I had purposely booked for its proximity to the race start. As we were checking in, I informed the concierge that I was running the marathon and inquired as to the best way to get to the race start. He suggested it would be easiest to take a taxi and that it would be unnecessary to reserve one in advance because there would be several waiting outside the hotel. Not reserving a taxi concerned me: the race started at 5 a.m. because of the heat, and I didn't want to run the risk of being left without a ride. But the concierge reassured me that there would indeed be a taxi waiting for me.

I woke up very early, having learned that a marathon start is not something that you want to cut close. Things can and will inevitably go wrong, and you will more often than not need extra time to deal with unforeseen occurrences. The concierge told me the night before that it should only take five to ten minutes to get to the race start, so I arrived in the lobby at 4:15 a.m. I was extremely relieved to see a taxi waiting outside for me.

A handful of runners were milling about as I hopped in the car. I told the driver that I needed to go to the marathon start, as if she couldn't guess this from my attire and the ungodly hour. She said no problem, and off we went.

It was pitch dark as we sped through the quiet streets. Throngs of runners shuffled down the sidewalks alongside us. As we passed through several police barricades, the driver informed me that some roads were closed and she would have to take a back route. "No problem," I replied. "I've got plenty of time." Down the deserted roads we flew and soon there were no more runners to be seen. A few more minutes passed and the trip was beginning to feel longer than necessary. Then the driver pulled over to the curb at a four-way intersection and announced that we had arrived. Due to the closed-off streets, she could go no further, but all I needed to do was walk down the street for a short way and I would be there. I paid her, said thanks, and exited the car.

The moment the door slammed and the taxi sped off, I knew something was wrong.

I was in a business district and there was not a soul in sight. I reassured myself that the driver knew where she was going; I was probably at a special back entrance to the race start. I began walking down the deserted street in the direction she had specified.

After a few minutes, it became increasingly apparent that something was not right. There were tens of thousands of participants in the marathon and I could not see or hear a soul. I broke into a fast jog and randomly made right and left turns in a vain attempt to find someone, anyone, to point me in the right direction.

After minutes that seemed like an hour, I saw two shadowy figures in the distance. As I ran toward them, I could see that one was on a ladder and the other was holding it steady. "Do you know where the marathon start is?" I asked, praying that it was right around the corner but suspecting that it couldn't possibly be. As the final word left my mouth, the man on the ladder turned to face me, and in his hands was a sign that read:

"Mile 2."

Not good.

He looked at me quizzically and pointed down the empty street.

"It's two miles that way."

Really not good.

I glanced at my watch. The time read 4:42 and my heart rate read 120. I could make it.

I thanked the man and took off into the darkness. I figured I would run eight-minute miles and arrive at the start line with a few minutes to spare. I passed the sign for Mile 1 at 4:50 a.m.; right on schedule. Slowly but surely I began to see other people on the sides of the road, and before long, I was running through the police escort motorcycles and cars, right to the front of the marathon start. The moment I stopped and turned around to face in the right direction, the sounds of the national anthem filled the air and a barrage of fireworks illuminated the Hawaiian sky. Less than one minute later, we were off.

EXPO

Most races hold an expo before the marathon. It may last one or more days and it is usually the place where you pick up your race number, timing chip (if they will be used), goodie bag, and T-shirt. Often you will receive a confirmation card in the mail that contains all your information. This is what you will need to pick up your number. Put the card in a safe place the moment it arrives and don't forget to bring it with you to the expo. Many marathons require a picture ID along with the confirmation card to pick up your bib number.

Some expos are small and some are quite large, depending on the marathon and the number of participants. There are usually vendor booths where you can find running-related goods and hear lectures on running topics. Although these booths sell a variety of running merchandise, do not assume that you will be able to buy your essential race items at the expo. They may run out of what you need or not carry it at all.

Many vendors give things away at the expo—a great way to get free **swag** and try a new product or two. These freebies include lots of nutritional items, such as new food and drink products, and runners walk up and down the aisles stuffing their faces with substances they have never consumed before. I urge you not to. You do not want to try anything new, much less a bunch of new things, the day before or even several days before your marathon. Take the freebies, but try them after your marathon, not before. You never know how you will react to new products, and you can jeopardize your race pretty fast with a seemingly innocuous sports bar or drink.

Swag, or Stuff We All Get: Free stuff, often given out at the expo and found in your race bag.

Don't spend hours upon hours at the expo, either. Remember that you have 26.2 miles to run, and standing for three hours the day before your marathon is not such a good idea. Go, have fun, pick up your bag, buy some gear, visit some booths, and then get off your feet.

FINAL STEPS

TEN COMMANDMENTS OF MARATHONING

1. Thou shall not try anything on race day that thee have not done in practice.

2. Thy first goal is always just to finish.

3. Thou shall drinketh at thine aid stations.

4. Thou shall not covet thy neighbor's marathon time.

5. It is not about thee who goes out the fastest; it's about thee who slows down the least.

6. Honor thy taper.

7. Carbs are thy best friend, not thine enemy.

8. Thou shall not believe that more is better.

9. Thou shall not skip thy strength training.

10. Thou shall stretch and stretch frequently.

THE DAY BEFORE THE RACE

I begin my carbo-loading and consume more salt four days before a marathon. I take in three to four carbohydrate drinks on each of the three days prior to the race, spreading them out throughout the day. If the race is on a Sunday, I begin this process on Thursday, and I suggest you do the same. You can either use carbohydrate drinks, such as Carbo Force, or take in more carbohydrate-rich foods. I find it much easier to take in my additional carbohydrates in liquid form and have had great success with this strategy. I take in a few salt tablets each day, eat salty foods that I normally avoid, such as pretzels, and drink sports drinks containing sodium.

I like to stretch more in the days leading up to a marathon, and I have a massage three or four days before the race. I don't like to get massaged too close to race day, but this is merely a personal preference. Some contend that it's good to have a massage close to your race, while others recommend against it. Do what works best for you. I wouldn't have a deep-tissue massage very close to race day, but again, if that seems to work for you, stick with it.

Two nights before the marathon is when you want a good night's sleep. This is the one that matters most, not the night before the race. Do not worry if you toss and turn the night before your marathon because this sleep is not essential to your performance, and most runners will be going on less sleep than they are used to. If you correctly tapered and rested until the last day before the race, that night's sleep is almost irrelevant.

The day before the marathon, you should have visited the expo and picked up your race bag and number. My system is to take the bag back to my room and dump the contents on the bed. I then separate the contents into three piles: things that I need for the race, a pile of swag I want to keep, and a pile of things I will throw away. If you follow my system, then throw the garbage pile into the trash, put aside the pile of sponsor swag, and add the race items to the rest of your race clothes and gear. If the marathon will be using a chip, put it on your race shoes immediately. Do the same with your race number.

The day before the marathon, you should run for ten minutes or so. I suggest this short session for two reasons: first, to release any last-minute stress and anxiety caused by your taper and the impending marathon, and second, to try out the exact clothes and gear you will wear in the marathon one last time. This means everything, including your race number. Don't be shy: either pin it on or put it on your race belt for a final test run. This step is especially impor-tant if you broke the first commandment of marathoning and plan to wear or use something for the first time during the race: It is your last chance to test it out during a short run. So go out in your race attire and gear, stretch your legs, blow off some steam, and then go back, take everything off, and put it in a neat pile. This way, when you wake up in the morning, everything is ready to go.

Some marathons have a pasta party either one or two nights before the race. These can be fun events, allowing you to meet other runners and psych yourself up for the race. The meal typically consists of a simple pasta and salad as one of your carbo-load pre-race dinners. Whether you attend this dinner is completely optional. Some runners love these events, but others find them stressful. It can be an easy way to take in some carbohydrates, but many runners would rather eat their own tried-and-true pre-race dinner. Wherever you decide to eat, just don't consume anything that you have never had before or a food that may disagree with you. In other words, this is probably not a good time to go to a Mexican restaurant, especially if you are not used to Mexican food.

If you are planning to use a system such as a Fuel Belt with gels and liquids, fill up your bottles the night before. You can put them in the refrigerator overnight to keep them cold, but be sure not to forget them. Make sure your empty belt is in your race pile and/or tape a note somewhere such as the bathroom mirror to remind you to bring these bottles with you.

The Day of the Race

Many races will give you a "baggage check" bag when you pick up your number and timing chip. It is usually a large plastic bag with your bib number on it that you can bring to the marathon start. You can use the bag to store any clothing, gear, and miscellaneous items that you bring to the marathon start as well as any items you wish to have immediately after the race; you will pick it up right after crossing the finish line. This bag is especially helpful at marathons where you arrive at the starting area early and spend considerable time, often a few hours, before the race actually begins. The New York City and Boston marathons are two races where you generally have to spend a good deal of time at the "athlete village" before the race start. You essentially set up a camp for yourself and just wait. One big mistake to avoid is getting cold while you are waiting. Your race clothing is usually minimal because your body will warm up as you run, but the outfit may be inadequate to keep you warm as you wait around before the race starts. Overdress to go to the start. Wear sweatpants and a sweatshirt or jacket. You can always remove these layers, but you will be miserable if you are freezing before you begin your 26.2-mile journey. These extra layers can serve a double function: Many marathons are considerably cooler at the finish, especially when you stop running. As you pick up your baggage check bag right after you finish, you can put the same clothes back on to keep you warm as your body temperature plummets. You will be very happy you have extra layers if it gets cold; trust me on this one.

You may also want a blanket to lie down on, plus food and drinks. Nutrition and hydration can be really important depending on when you eat breakfast and the time your race starts. You don't want to go for several hours without eating or drinking before your marathon, and many times this can be the case. So, in addition to wearing several extra layers to the start of your marathon to keep yourself warm both before and after the race, bring extra food and beverages to ensure that you are properly hydrated and your fuel stores are adequately topped off. What and how much you take in is highly individualized and should mimic what you consumed before training runs. Eat a tried-and-true breakfast on race morning, and then be sure to eat and drink again roughly two hours later. You want to take in some good carbs, such as a bagel, a gel, or an energy bar. Hydrate as well, drinking at least eight to ten ounces of a beverage twenty minutes or so before the start. Consuming a sports drink such as Gatorade can serve both purposes because it will hydrate you while supplying carbohydrates.

As I discussed earlier, I believe that re-fueling is critically important right after hard workouts, and never is this more true than immediately after you run a marathon. For this reason, I put recovery drinks into my baggage check bag so that I can consume them in the minutes after I finish my race. For the majority of runners, myself included, eating or drinking is usually the last thing we feel like doing after a race. Our stomachs are upset and we really don't want to take in anything. Well, I force myself. I typically have a bottle of water, a bottle of Gatorade, a car-bohydrate/protein drink such as Endurox that I have mixed together beforehand, and a Myoplex shake. I take in all of these within a few minutes after the race, replenishing my glycogen stores with carbohydrates, in-gesting protein to help rebuild my damaged muscles, rehydrating with water, and replac-ing lost electrolytes with Gatorade. You should consider doing so as well to optimize your recovery.

I also bring my MP3 player, because I love to listen to music as close to the race start as possible. When I have to lie around and wait for a while, I like listening to mu-sic as I do my relaxation and visualization exercises.

Note: Can you listen to music during a race? Check your marathon's rules. Certain races prohibit listening to portable music devices; others state that it is illegal, but race officials look the other way when runners use them.

I have a disposable camera to take pic-tures of family, friends, and other marathon sights before the race starts. I pack a cell phone so that I can easily locate the people who will be waiting for me at the finish line. I have my Bodyglide to apply another coat of antifriction gel minutes before the race begins (I apply the first coat as I dress in the morning), and I also have sunscreen. I bring my food and drinks, having packed them in a separate plastic bag in case they leak. And yes, I bring toilet paper, the equivalent of gold at the start of a marathon.

Note: The grand spectacle of rows upon rows of portable toilets at the staging area of the larger marathons is only overshadowed by the sheer number of runners lined up to use them. Regardless of the size of your marathon, you will undoubtedly have to use a portable toilet at least once, most likely twice, depending upon how early you arrive at the start. I recommend getting in line as soon as you arrive and again twenty minutes or so before the race start. The lines can creep along at a snail's pace, and you don't want to be twenty-fifth in line with five minutes until race start. Also, when you finally get to use one, there is typically no toilet paper. Since you're already dragging your baggage check bag around, just throw in some tissues or a small roll of toilet paper. Just be warned that toilet paper can be such a rare commodity that runners will swarm whomever has some.

If it is cool at the race start, it might be wise to wear a "throwaway" shirt. This is an old shirt that you wear to keep warm and then you literally throw it away at some point during the race. Many people wear these layers into the start corrals and then fling them off to the side right before the race starts. Old race shirts are great for this purpose, especially long-sleeve shirts. Many races will donate this discarded clothing to charity. Other runners may choose to keep this layer on for a few miles and then discard it at a water station once they have warmed up. If the race is significantly colder at the start, you can choose to wear throwaway sweats, hats, and gloves as well. If you wear extra layers at the start of your race, it is always a good idea to choose items that you can throw away if need be, so choose clothes that you are not overly attached to.

Note: Some runners buy inexpensive gloves, such as painter's gloves, to keep their hands warm at the start and then toss them during the marathon. You can also find inexpensive gloves that are perfect for this purpose at many expos. You don't have to throw them away because they are usually small enough to tuck away somewhere.

MARATHON CHECKLIST

- [ ] 1. Running shoes
- [ ] 2. Bib number
- [ ] 3. Timing chip (if one will be used)
- [ ] 4. Race shorts/pants
- [ ] 5. Race shirt
- [ ] 6. Bib number belt or pins
- [ ] 7. Sweat pants
- [ ] 8. Sweatshirt
- [ ] 9. Throwaway shirt
- [ ] 10. Hat/visor
- [ ] 11. Sunglasses
- [ ] 12. Running watch
- [ ] 13. Gloves/throwaway gloves
- [ ] 14. Gels
- [ ] 15. Fuel Belt
- [ ] 16. Bodyglide/Vaseline
- [ ] 17. Marker (to write name on shirt or arms)
- [ ] 18. Food/drink to consume before the start of the race
- [ ] 19. Toilet paper
- [ ] 20. Disposable camera
- [ ] 21. Blanket
- [ ] 22. Sunscreen
- [ ] 23. Cell phone
- [ ] 24. *Your excuse:* Tim, a phenomenal runner and relative of mine, never leaves home for a marathon without his excuse. When you ask him on race morning how he's feeling, he'll moan, "My back's really sore," or, "I think I'm coming down with a cold," laying the groundwork ahead of time so he has somewhere to place the blame if he falls short of his goal. It's a sound strategy that you may want to consider, especially if you are racing against a family member, friend, or coworker.

CHAPTER 8
The Marathon

You should arrive at the start with plenty of time to spare just in case a last-minute issue arises, because it almost always does. If you have a baggage check bag, drop it off at a designated area on your way to the start. Even this can take time, so don't cut it too close. Assume that everything you need to do before the race will take much longer than expected, and you will avoid major potential stress.

Find your designated corral, if you are at a big marathon, and line up. At the smaller marathons that do not have corrals there are usually signs indicating where you should line up based on your pace. So if you plan on running a ten-minute pace, find the appropriate sign and join the runners in that section. Do not make the common mistake of lining up with a group significantly faster than your pace. If you hope to average nine minutes per mile, do not jump in with the seven-minute-per-mile runners. You may think this would be to your advantage, but

it is a big mistake. You will be forced to run much faster than you want at the start—a problem even when you line up with the correct group—but by joining a faster group, you will push the early pace even more. This can be disastrous in a marathon. In addition, you will suffer mentally as throngs of runners hammer past you for several miles. You can get pushed around and even knocked down in these situations, so please don't make this mistake. It is a very bad way to begin a race that you have trained so hard for.

Once the starting gun goes off, the fun begins. Don't worry about how far back you are from the starting line. If you have a timing chip, your race won't begin until you cross that line. Nor should you be concerned if the crowds ahead of you are keeping you from running as fast as you'd like early on. Consider it a blessing. This will force you to run conservatively at the start rather than shooting out too fast. Running one to two minutes slower per mile for the first few miles is just fine; running thirty seconds too fast spells big trouble.

Moreover, once the gun goes off, you will likely need to use the bathroom again. It doesn't matter if you went right before lining up; it just happens to be the way the body works. Take the time to go.

Note: Many runners refuse to slow down or stop for even a moment during a marathon. Take the time to go to the bathroom, tie a loose shoelace, pick up a PowerGel you dropped, or stop at an aid station to rub Vaseline on a hot spot. By taking these few extra seconds, you will most likely end up running faster, not slower. Running twenty miles with a full bladder is not a heck of a lot of fun and will slow you down much more than the time it takes to use the bathroom.

WELCOME TO THE PARTY

Try to let go of all the stress and anxiety that you have been feeling up until this moment. This is the party; this is why you logged so many miles and did so many crunches. If you put in the training and set appropriate goals for yourself, you should feel great. Enjoy every moment. You have worked too hard not to enjoy the fruits of you labor.

For the first few miles, focus on holding your pace where it should be, slow and steady. When in doubt, go slower. You will probably be shocked when you pass the first several mile markers. Chances are you will be running much faster than you thought, but it will feel surprisingly easy. You can't believe how fast you are going and that you are on track to finish ahead of what you had expected.

Remember my earlier lesson about being on track? Never forget it.

You didn't morph overnight from a nine-minute-per-mile runner into an eight-minute-per-mile runner. My training plans are good, but not that good. Slow down.

Note: At each mile marker, most races have either digital clocks showing the running time or volunteers calling out the time as you pass.

Take in the sights and sounds as you let your body warm up. Perform frequent body checks and stretches early on. Do not, under any circumstances, skip the water stations. Bigger races will have water stops on both sides of the road to ease congestion, while smaller races may have them on just one side. At a larger race with aid stations on both sides of the road, you will see a station on one side first, and when that one ends, a station on the opposite side begins. Water is commonly offered first, followed by a sports drink toward the end.

As you approach the water stop, gradually slow down. Look over your shoulder and see whether there are any runners close to you. Be very careful at these stops; runners ahead of you will often come to a dead stop with no warning, while runners behind you can crash into you as they focus on grabbing a drink and not those around them. Volunteers hold out cups with extended arms. I like to make eye contact with the volunteer whose cup I am going to take and point to it as well. This way they know I am coming and they can begin to move toward me.

Get your cup and move through the aid station area. The longer you remain in the area, the greater your chances of getting slammed into. I like to get past the station and move to the side of the road. I then slow down to a fast walk and take in my fluids along with any salt tablets or PowerGels. These four or five extra seconds will ensure that I take in what I need; then I am off and running again.

If you insist on running with your fluid, first dump some out on the road if it is filled to the top. Pinch the top until there are two flat sides to the cup and place one of the corners into your mouth. This directs the majority of the fluid into your mouth and not down the front of your shirt.

If it is a particularly hot day, I will grab an extra cup of water to dump on my head. This helps keep my core body temperature down and may prevent me from overheating. When I have slowed to a fast walk past the aid station, I dump the water over my head, drink my Gatorade and/or water, and off I go.

Note: If you want to dump water over your head (and I encourage you to do so), just make sure you're holding water and not a sports drink. Many runners make this mistake and it's not a great feeling to be covered in a sticky, sugary solution for miles on end.

If you miss a water station because you didn't get over in time, I suggest that you move to the side and make your way back. Volunteers will often see you coming and run to you with a drink. Do not skip the fluids; they are vital to your success.

Note: Be courteous to the volunteers along the course. They are just that: volunteers. They donate their time so that you can have a great race. They are doing their best and things can and will go wrong. Do not take anything out on them. Treat them with respect and thank them every chance you get.

Stick to the nutrition and hydration plan you have practiced for weeks. Take in your food and fluids. Remember that you may feel queasy at times, but I will take queasy over dehydrated or bonking any day of the week. You can use mental tools to tough it out during stomach distress, but they won't work if you have become dehydrated or your glycogen levels are depleted.

When you hit the half-marathon point, you should continue to exercise restraint. If you are feeling great, that's terrific, but it does not mean you should "put down the hammer" and drastically pick up your pace. There is still plenty of serious running left. If you are an experienced runner who is good at judging your pace, you can increase it slightly, but don't push too hard too soon. And if you are feeling poorly and are behind schedule, don't get down on yourself. One of the characteristics of endurance racing is the incredible roller coaster of highs and lows. Just because you feel bad one minute does not mean you will feel the same way in five minutes. Use self-talk to pull yourself out of your current mind-set and to change the way you feel physically. Try every mental tool available to push yourself through the rough patch. Put a smile on your face.

> **Note:** I'm not sure who said it, but here's a fantastic line that's so applicable to marathon running: "When you are feeling bad, put a smile on your face. When it hurts too much to smile, slow down."

MY LAS VEGAS MARATHON EXPERIENCE

The Las Vegas Marathon really showed me the highs and lows associated with running a marathon. It was my first true lesson that you can never give up, that you may feel horrible one moment and fantastic the next, and that this back and forth can continue throughout the marathon. The key is to stay positive and keep moving forward.

It was the first year I was trying to qualify for the Boston Marathon, and I needed a sub-3:10. I ran a 3:19 at the New York City Marathon and a 3:12 in Philadelphia several weeks later. Determined to run Boston that year, I traveled to Las Vegas to make one more attempt.

The whole experience seemed doomed from the very start. I needed to take an all-day fitness certification test the day before departing, and I had to take a very late flight that would arrive in Vegas after midnight. I took the test and jumped on the plane. I thought I would catch some much-needed sleep, but the guy next to me talked the entire flight.

I arrived in Vegas and got to the hotel and to sleep well after midnight, only to get up a few hours later to board the bus for the desert. (This was the "old" Las Vegas Marathon; I believe the new one starts and finishes downtown.) We were packed into school buses that were neither comfortable nor warm. We arrived in the middle of the desert in the predawn dark, and I tried to catch some sleep in the back of the bus before the race start.

I may have slept for ten minutes, and then it was time to run. Needless to say, I wasn't in the best frame of mind. As we ran the first mile, my body felt terrible: My legs felt like lead, and I thought, There is no way this is happening today. When I hit the first mile marker and the clock read 7:58, my dreams of Boston began to fade. I needed to average 7:15s to run under 3:10. The next few miles were the same; each clock registered around eight-minute miles. I stopped for a long bathroom break at mile six and figured I was now in it just to finish.

As I left the Porta-potty and began to run again, I started to feel better. The sun was rising and the air became warmer. I could feel that I was picking up the pace and my effort level seemed to be falling. When I reached the half-marathon point, I was still not on track to break 3:10, but I was feeling strong and thought, Let's just see what I can do. I picked up the pace and relied on mental techniques to push myself faster.

When I hit the twenty-mile mark, I was deep in the zone for the first time in my life. My endorphins had kicked in and, although I was definitely pushing the pace and suffering, it was not unbearable. A few miles later, I checked my watch and did some quick math: If I picked it up a little more, there was a remote chance I could reach my goal. I would have to hold a pace that I had never before run in a marathon, but I told myself I could suffer for three miles for the chance of qualifying for Boston. I passed more and more people, which increased my confidence and pace even more. As I hit the twenty-five-mile marker, I put the hammer down and began my kick to the finish. My lungs and legs were screaming but I told myself I could hold it for just a few minutes longer.

I crossed the finish line in 3:09:41.

That Las Vegas race taught me that the old clichés are true: Never give up, and it's not over until it's over. Don't ever give up during your marathon, no matter how bad you feel. It's a long race, and things can and will change. You are much stronger than you think, and you can push your body far beyond what you believe are your limitations.

Try to stay "in the moment" throughout your marathon: Don't focus on what lies ahead but rather on how you feel right then and there. I like to approach a marathon as twenty-six one-mile races, and if you ask me during the course what mile I am on, I might not know. I am never thinking, "I have ten miles to go," but rather, "I feel great right now." My goal is to get to the next mile marker, one by one. If you need to break up the marathon in a different way, you can also try dividing it into four separate parts: up to mile six, then the half-marathon, up to mile twenty, and then the final six to the finish.

MILE TWENTY AND BEYOND

If you are going to run into trouble, chances are you will feel it around mile twenty. If you carbohydrate-loaded sufficiently and did your long runs, you should have no major problems at this point other than general fatigue. You will understand how the race really starts at mile twenty because many runners failed to do one or both of these correctly, and you will see the suffering kick in at this point.

Note: Make sure your bib number is visible throughout your marathon if you wish to buy pictures of yourself afterward. Most races have photographers stationed at specific points along the course; they snap thousands of pictures and sort them by bib number. This goes for the finish as well; make sure your number is clearly visible as you approach the finish line if you wish to have photographic proof of your accomplishment.

Even if you fueled up and trained correctly, the final miles will still be challenging. Stay strong; this is definitely the time you want to engage in intensive self-talk. Think back to all the work you did for the race and how nervous you were beforehand. If you are on track for your goal, let that realization make you even stronger. If you have run into difficulties and are off track, put a big smile on your face and remember that the primary goal is to finish. No matter what the outcome of your marathon, the bottom line is that you took on a challenge and set about achieving it. The best thing that comes of missing your goal is that you probably got into the best shape of your life and learned exactly what you are made of. Does it really matter that you ran a 4:20 but wanted to go under four hours? There is no failure when it comes to running a marathon—only lessons learned and the "next time."

Even though I have run dozens upon dozens of marathons around the world, I get choked up every time I cross the finish line. It is an indescribable experience to challenge yourself physically and push beyond your perceived limits. When you cross that finish line—and you will—know that you have accomplished something to be extremely proud of, regardless of what the clock reads.

THE GALLOWAY METHOD

Former Olympian and current running guru Jeff Galloway introduced his run/walk strategy to thousands of runners, and you will see hundreds of his converts at most every marathon. Built on periodic structured walk breaks, Galloway's method has enabled more people run marathons, to run injury free, and, believe it or not, run faster.

. Many running purists argue that if you walk during a marathon, you are not a true runner. Oh, really? I thought that it was a race, and that the rules state that you can run, walk, or crawl to the finish, and the first one to do so wins.

A primary goal of any great coach is to find ways to improve performance with less work, both in training and while racing. Taking walk breaks does both when it comes to marathon running. Remember when I said that running a marathon is not about who goes the fastest but who slows down the least? Walk breaks help keep you from slowing down as the marathon progresses. I know because I have tried Galloway's method with fantastic results.

The first time I ran a sub-3:00 marathon, I used the Galloway method. It happened at the Chicago Marathon, and if you are not familiar with the course, it is extremely flat and extremely fast. (It is also a fantastic place to set a PR and to try to qualify for the Boston Marathon, if that is one of your goals.) My goal was to run just under three hours, averaging 6:50s for a 2:59 finish.

My strategy was to take ten-second walk breaks every mile for the first thirteen miles; at the halfway point, I would assess my pace and how I was feeling to see whether I would continue with the plan.

Note: I believe that if walk breaks are to work, they must start at mile one. If you begin using them at mile six or mile ten, it's too late. Beginning walk breaks early on, when the majority of runners are hammering way too fast, takes a great deal of discipline but pays huge dividends in the end.

At every mile marker, I took a walk break of ten seconds. I moved way over to one side of the road, slowed to a fast walk, then started right back up again. I was averaging seven minutes per mile for the first ten miles or so. When I arrived at the half-marathon point, my time was 1:31:35, putting me on track for a 3:03 or slightly slower. I felt fantastic and decided to stop the walk breaks and push the pace.

I was amazed that at around mile twenty, I began to pass people with ease. Because it is my practice to run negative splits, passing people in the later miles of a marathon is not new to me. But what was new on that day was how strong I felt; in fact, I had never felt better and I was holding the fastest pace I had ever run. Long story short, I ended up running a 2:59:44. Mission accomplished, and I did it using walk breaks.

I also rely on walk breaks when I pace certain clients during marathons. The frequency and length of the walk breaks will vary greatly depending on the client's fitness level, the race conditions, and our goals. I ran the Big Sur (California) Marathon with my dad utilizing Galloway's method. My father was sixty at the time, and the trip was my birthday gift to him. He had just run the Boston Marathon, so this would be his second marathon in six days. I had him take a full-minute walk break every mile and we ended up running a 4:43 on the extremely hilly course. Not too shabby for an old guy.

I will not discuss the physiology of why these walk breaks may work; let me just say that, based on my results and the results of my clients, they just do. But don't take my word for it; try it by experimenting with walk breaks to see how they work for you. Many people ask whether it's necessary to do them in training. I did not while training for my first sub-3 marathon, so I don't believe you have to practice them to be successful. That said, I do use them when training certain clients by incorporating them into longer runs. These tend to be unstructured breaks, however, and not necessarily every mile. I choose to do this for no other reason than I believe taking walk breaks during training runs will help many people avoid injury.

Although there is no hard-and-fast rule dictating how frequently you should take walk breaks and for how long, I recommend the following:

- 5- to 6-hour marathoners: A 1-minute walk break every mile.

- 4- to 5-hour marathoners: 30- to 60-second walk breaks every mile.

- 3- to 4-hour marathoners: A 10-second walk break every mile.

- Under 3-hour marathoners: 10-second walk breaks every mile with the option of stopping the breaks at any mile after mile 13.

PACE GROUPS

Many marathons offer pace groups that you can sign up for, usually at the expo. Led by an experienced runner who can hold a specific pace, these groups can help you achieve your desired time goal. They are usually broken up into groups such as 5:00, 4:30, 4:00, 3:30, 3:15, 3:00, and so on. The leader may carry a sign announcing the time goal, and group members may also wear a piece of paper on their backs showing the time. Participation in these groups is usually free, and keeping up with your group guarantees that you will hit your time. There is power in numbers, and having someone who runs an accurate and steady pace can really help. If this interests you, inquire about pace groups at the expo information booth.

Marathon Pace Chart

Mile Pace	Finish Time
4:45	2:04:32
5:00	2:11:06
5:15	2:17:39
5:30	2:24:12
5:45	2:30:45
6:00	2:37:19
6:15	2:43:52
6:30	2:50:25
6:45	2:56:59
7:00	3:03:32
7:15	3:10:05
7:30	3:16:38
7:45	3:23:12
8:00	3:29:45
8:15	3:36:18
8:30	3:42:52
8:45	3:49:25
9:00	3:55:58
9:15	4:02:31
9:30	4:09:05
9:45	4:15:38
10:00	4:22:11
10:30	4:35:18
11:00	4:48:24
11:30	5:01:31
12:00	5:14:37

Source: www.marathonguide.com

"RUNNING THE TANGENTS"

I am struck by how few runners understand the concept and take advantage of "running the tangents." It means running the shortest distance between two points and using the entire width of the road to your advantage. Although some people incorrectly consider this cheating, it is actually how race organizers measure the course. In effect, you want to "cut corners," so staying on one side of the road for the whole race is not the way to go unless the course is a perfectly straight line from start to finish. For example, if the course has a curve to the left, you would start the curve on the right side of the road, gradually crossing over the middle through the turn, and finishing on the left side. For an S-shaped turn, you would try to straighten it out as much as possible instead of running on the same side through each twist and turn. Running the tangents is not always possible when running in a crowd, but you should take advantage of this strategy whenever you can. A marathon is long enough and you do not want to run any farther than you have to.

> **Note:** In a particularly curvy course, the time you save running the tangents can really add up. There is also a mental boost that comes from passing runners by relying on this strategy.

RUNNING WITH A FRIEND

Many people find that training for a marathon with a friend is a great motivator. They may even decide to run the marathon together. Be careful if you decide to do this. The marathon experience can be quite different from short training runs, and all of a sudden, running with another person becomes a problem. One of you might not feel well at mile twenty and want to stop or even quit, leaving the partner with the dilemma of whether to stay with or separate from the running mate. Sometimes it's simply that one partner is better trained than the other and wants to take off instead of holding the slower pace with the friend. Whatever the case may be, make sure you clearly discuss beforehand what you will do if and when such a situation arises. Will you stick together through thick and thin, or will one run ahead? And, if one runs ahead, will the other feel resentful? I recommend making a pact that if it looks like you need to split up, then do so with no hard feelings. Try to stay together as long as possible, but as soon as it becomes problematic, each of you is on your own.

CHAPTER 9
Post-Marathon

After your marathon, you need to take time off, both to savor your accomplishment and to let your body rest and recover. I recommend at least several days of complete relaxation post-race. You might want to schedule a massage for the following one or two days as well. You may be very sore and that is to be expected. Both beginners as well as veteran runners who run fast will experience post-marathon soreness. You may have significant difficulty going up and down stairs and even standing and sitting. I actually enjoy this post-marathon soreness in a twisted sort of way! Rest assured that it will pass. After a few days, you can slowly resume exercising to help you loosen up. You can engage in cross-training activities such as bike riding or swimming, or you can go out for a short, easy run.

Take time to reflect upon your achievement, whether it is your first marathon or your fortieth. Review your training notes and see where you can make improvements.

Run your marathon again in your mind and see what you would change next time and what you think really worked this time. Re-evaluate the goals that you set for yourself. Realize that you have accomplished an incredible feat; it may seem like everyone has run a marathon, but you actually belong to a select group. Be thankful that you are healthy enough to run and don't ever take it for granted. And, after you have done all this, start looking into your next marathon!

PMS: POST-MARATHON SYNDROME

Many runners, myself included, experience what I refer to as PMS, or post-marathon syndrome. It is a form of depression that comes soon after your marathon day. It is a natural response, and it's easy to understand its etiology: You devoted a significant part of your life to a single purpose and now that you have achieved it, there is a feeling of sadness or letdown. (This seems to be true whether you achieved or fell short of your goal.) I believe the reaction stems from having a definitive purpose, and it illustrates the power of goal setting. This is just one reason I love marathons: They give us direction and a goal to reach for and they compel us to engage in healthy habits to achieve that goal. So, after you have taken time to reflect on your marathon experience and allowed your body to recover, start looking into your next event. It need not be another marathon or even a long running race, for that matter. It can be a triathlon, an organized bike ride, an adventure race, or a shorter-distance run-

ning race such as a 5K or 10K. The point is to stay active while giving yourself a clear goal to shoot for. This will surely cure your PMS and get you back on track.

Below you will find 16-week marathon (and half-marathon) training plans for beginners, intermediate, and advanced levels. For further explanation of the tables' content, see chapter 5.

How much time do you need between marathons? I love when I see formulas purporting to answer this question. There is simply no universal response. Some people can run one marathon per year; others can

THE FINISH LINE

I love running. I run for my head, for my body, and for my life. I am thankful for every day that I am healthy enough to put on running shoes and head out the door. I love running by myself; with my wife, Philippa; with my dad; and with my Labrador, Lucy; and I can't wait to start running with my new son, Tommy. Thank you for purchasing my book and trying my plans and advice. I promise that if you follow these guidelines and apply them consistently, you will become the best runner you can be. You will also enjoy your running more than ever before. I look forward to seeing you at the races; I'll be the one running with a big smile on my face.

Push your limits and experience what happens when we accomplish what we didn't dream was possible.

Believe in yourself.

run fifty or more. It is highly individualistic and there is a list of factors to consider, including your fitness level, years of running experience, goals, cross-training and strength-training habits, running pace, and more. It seems that the slower you run, the less recovery your body may need and the more races you can do. Remember that my sixty-year-old father ran two marathons in less than a week and plans to do so again. He is not Superman, but he has been running for well over thirty years and has learned what is needed for longevity in running. The answer depends on knowing and listening to your body. The more races you wish to do, the more paramount your consistency in strength training, flexibility, nutrition, and hydration become. Remember that running should primarily be about health; don't try to compile a list of marathon finishes at your body's expense. The goal should be to run into your nineties and beyond.

Appendix A

Below you will find 16-week marathon (and half-marathon) training plans for beginner, intermediate, and advanced levels. For further explanation of the tables, see chapter 5. The "down" weeks and taper phase are shaded gray.

Beginner Half-Marathon Plan

Week	Mon	Tues	Wed	Thurs	Fri	Sat	Sun	Total
16	OFF	3	weights	3	weights	3	3	12
15	OFF	3	weights	3	weights	3	3	12
14	OFF	3	weights	4	weights	3	4	14
13	OFF	3	weights	4	weights	3	4	14
12	OFF	3	weights	3	weights	3	3	12
11	OFF	3	weights	4	weights	3	5	15
10	OFF	4	weights	5	weights	3	6	18
9	OFF	4	weights	4	weights	3	4	15
8	OFF	4	weights	5	weights	3	7	19
7	OFF	4	weights	4	weights	3	9	20
6	OFF	3	weights	4	weights	3	5	15
5	OFF	4	weights	5	weights	3	10	22
4	OFF	5	weights	6	weights	3	11	25
3	OFF	3	OFF	5	OFF	4	6	18
2	OFF	3	OFF	5	OFF	3	4	15
1	OFF	4	OFF	3	OFF	10 min	RACE	

Beginner Marathon Plan

Week	Mon	Tues	Wed	Thurs	Fri	Sat	Sun	Total
16	OFF	3	weights	4	weights	3	6	16
15	OFF	3	weights	4	weights	3	6	16
14	OFF	4	weights	5	weights	4	6	19
13	OFF	4	weights	5	weights	4	8	21
12	OFF	4	weights	5	weights	4	10	23
11	OFF	4	weights	6	weights	3	11	24
10	OFF	4	weights	6	weights	3	13	26
9	OFF	4	weights	5	weights	3	8	20
8	OFF	4	weights	5	weights	4	14	27
7	OFF	4	weights	6	weights	3	16	29
6	OFF	3	weights	4	weights	3	13	23
5	OFF	4	weights	4	weights	4	18	30
4	OFF	3	weights	7	weights	OFF	20	30
3	OFF	4	OFF	6	OFF	4	8	22
2	OFF	3	OFF	5	OFF	3	6	17
1	OFF	4	OFF	3	OFF	10 min	RACE	

Intermediate Half Marathon Plan

Week	Mon	Tues	Wed	Thurs	Fri	Sat	Sun	Total
16	OFF	4	weights	5	weights	3 w/C	6	18
15	OFF	4	weights	5	weights	3 w/C	6	18
14	OFF	4	weights	5	weights	4 w/C	7	20
13	OFF	4	weights	5	weights	4 w/C	7	20
12	OFF	3	weights	5	weights	3 w/C	5	16
11	OFF	5	weights	6	weights	4 w/C	8	23
10	OFF	5	weights	6	weights	5 w/C	9	25
9	OFF	4	weights	6	weights	4 w/C	6	20
8	OFF	5	weights	6	weights	4 w/C	10	25
7	OFF	5	weights	6	weights	5 w/C	11	27
6	OFF	5	weights	6	weights	4 w/C	8	23
5	OFF	6	weights	6	weights	4 w/C	11	27
4	OFF	6	weights	6	weights	5 w/C	12	29
3	OFF	4	C	5	C	4	8	21
2	OFF	3	C	5	C	3	5	16
1	OFF	4	OFF	3	OFF	10 min	RACE	

C = core workout   w/C = with core workout

Intermediate Marathon Plan

Week	Mon	Tues	Wed	Thurs	Fri	Sat	Sun	Total
16	OFF	4	weights	4	weights	3 w/C	8	19
15	OFF	4	weights	5	weights	4 w/C	8	21
14	OFF	4	weights	5	weights	4 w/C	10	23
13	OFF	4	weights	5	weights	4 w/C	12	25
12	OFF	4	weights	4	weights	4 w/C	9 w/C	21
11	OFF	5	weights	6	weights	4 w/C	13	28
10	OFF	5	weights	6	weights	4 w/C	15	30
9	OFF	4	weights	5	weights	3 w/C	12	24
8	OFF	6	weights	6	weights	4 w/C	16	32
7	OFF	6	weights	7	weights	5 w/C	20	38
6	OFF	4	weights	8	weights	4 w/C	14	30
5	OFF	6	weights	8	weights	6 w/C	18	38
4	OFF	7	weights	10	weights	3 w/C	20	40
3	OFF	5	C	7	C	6	10	28
2	OFF	4	C	6	C	4	6	20
1	OFF	4	C	3	OFF	10 min	RACE	

C = core workout   w/C = with core workout

Advanced Half Marathon Plan

Week	Mon	Tues	Wed	Thurs	Fri	Sat	Sun	Total
16	0	4	W	6	W	4	6	20
15	0	4	W	6	W	4	6	20
14	0	4	W	6	W	5	8	23
13	0	4	W	6	W	5	8	23
12	0	4 w/3x3 min @ 1 min	W	5 w/6x30 sec HR	W	4 w/10 min T & C	6	19
11	0	5 w/3x3 min @ 1 min	W	6 w/6x30 sec HR	W	5 w/10 min T & C	9	25
10	0	5 w/3x3 min @ 1 min	W	6 w/6x30 sec HR	W	5 w/10 min T & C	11	27
9	0	5 w/7 min fartleks	W	6	W	4	7	22
8	0	5 w/5x3 min @ 1 min	W	6 w/6x1 min HR	W	5 w/15 min T & C	10	26
7	0	5 w/5x3 min @ 1 min	W	6 w/6x1 min HR	W	5 w/15 min T & C	12	28
6	0	4 w/5 min fartleks	W	5	W	4	8	21
5	0	6 w/2x5 min @ 2 min	W	6 w/6x1 min HR	W	5 w/15 min T & C	10	27
4	0	6 w/3x5 min @ 2 min	W	6 w/6x1 min HR	W	6 w/15 min T & C	12	30
3	0	5 w/5x2 min @ 1 min	O	5 w/6x30 sec HR	O	4 w/10 min T	7	21
2	0	4 w/5x1 min @ 1 min	O	4	O	3	5	16
1	0	4	O	3	O	10 min	RACE	

HR = hill repeats C = core workout W = weight routine O = Off T = Tempo

i.e., 4 w/3x3 min @ 1 min = 4 miles with 3 intervals of 3 minutes at 5K pace with 1 minute rest in between (easy jog).

i.e., 5 w/6x30 sec HR = 5 miles with 6 hill repeats of 30 seconds each. Jog or walk slowly back down to recover.

i.e., 5 w/10 min T & C = 5 miles with a 10-minute tempo at 10K pace plus core workout.

Advanced Marathon Plan

Week	Mon	Tues	Wed	Thurs	Fri	Sat	Sun	Total
16	0	5/C	W	6	4/C	4/C	10	25
15	0	5/C	W	6	4/C	4/C	13	28
14	0	5/C	W	6	4/C	4/C	15	30
13	0	4/C	W	5	W	3/C	9	21
12	0	6 w/3x5 min @ 2 min & C	W	8 w/6x30 sec HR	W	5 w/15 min T & C	14	33
11	0	6 w/3x5 min @ 2 min & C	W	8 w/6x30 sec HR	W	5 w/15 min T & C	20	39
10	0	6 w/10 min fartleks & C	W	8	W	4/C	12	30
9	0	8 w/4x5 min @ 2 min & C	W	10 w/6x1 min HR	W	6 w/20 min T & C	16	40
8	0	8 w/4x5 min @ 2 min & C	W	13 w/6x1 min HR	W	6 w/20 min T & C	20	47
7	0	8 w/10 min fartleks & C	W	10	W	4/C	13	35
6	0	9 w/6x5 min @ 2 min & C	W	10 w/6x1 min HR	W	7 w/25 min T & C	16	42
5	0	9 w/6x5 min @ 2 min & C	W	13 w/6x1 min HR	W	7 w/25 min T & C	18	47
4	0	10 w/6x5 min @ 2 min & C	W	13 w/6x1 min HR	W	7 w/25 min T & C	20	50
3	0	6 w/5x2 min @ 1 min & C	C	8 w/6x30 sec HR	C	6 w/20 min T & C	10	30
2	0	5 w/5x2 min @ 1 min & C	C	6	C	4 w/10 min T & C	8	23
1	0	6 w/5x1 min @ 1 min	0	3	0	10 min	RACE	

HR = hill repeats   C = core workout   W = weight routine   O = Off

i.e., 6 w/3x5 min @ 2 min & C = 6 miles with 3 intervals of 5 minutes at 5K pace with 2 minutes rest in between (easy jog) plus core workout.

i.e., 10 w/6x1 min HR = 10 miles with 6 hill repeats of 1 minute each. Jog or walk slowly back down to recover.

i.e., 6 w/20 min T & C = 6 miles with a 20-minute tempo at 10K pace plus core workout.

Marathon Goals Checklist

Outcome Goals:

1. _____
2. _____
3. _____

Performance Goals:

1. _____
2. _____
3. _____
4. _____
5. _____
6. _____
7. _____
8. _____
9. _____
10. _____

Process Goals:

1. _____
2. _____
3. _____
4. _____
5. _____
6. _____
7. _____
8. _____
9. _____
10. _____

RECOMMENDED WEBSITES

www.active.com
Online registration, calculators, and training advice.

www.aims-association.org
Association of International Marathons; includes a calendar.

www.americanrunning.org
Website of American Running Association; great fitness articles.

www.american-trackandfield.com
American Track and Field website.

www.bostonmarathon.org
Website for the Boston Marathon.

www.coolrunning.com
U.S. marathon and half marathon calendars, international marathon and half marathon calendars, marathon training, marathon news, running clubs, calculators, articles, and results.

www.fuelbelt.com
Hydration belts, packs, and more.

www.headsweats.com
Performance headwear.

www.jeffgalloway.com
Coaching, camps, and more.

www.marathon411.com
U.S. marathon and half marathon calendars, international marathon and half marathon calendars, marathon training, marathon news, and running clubs.

www.marathonguide.com
U.S. marathon and half marathon calendars, international marathon and half marathon calendar, marathon training, marathon news, running clubs, calculators, and articles.

www.marathontours.com
Marathon tour company providing entry, flight reservations, and accommodation services for numerous marathons.

www.nyrrc.org
Website for the New York Road Runner's Club; information on races in New York City and the New York City Marathon.

www.race360.com
Comprehensive online race calendar.

www.rrca.org
Race calendar, coaching, articles, and gear.

www.runnersworld.com
Comprehensive website of *Runner's World*
magazine.

www.runningnetwork.com
Race calendar, news, training tips,
and results.

www.runningtimes.com
Comprehensive website of *Running Times*
magazine.

www.teamholland.com
Fitness videos and books, fitness apparel,
coaching, camps, and fitness radio show
and Podcasts.

www.tn-sunglasses.us
Performance sunglasses.

www.usatf.org
U.S.A. Track and Field website.

ACKNOWLEDGMENTS

I would like to thank my wife Philippa for not only allowing me to run all over the world, but encouraging me to do so.

Thanks, Dad, for taking me along on your early marathon training runs and introducing me to the world of running. Thanks, Mom, for playing the Italian mother and overfeeding me afterwards.

Special thanks to race director extraordinaire Jim Gerwick; Dave Watt and the American Medical Athletic Association; PR gurus Melissa McNeese and Leslie McClure; and Cathy Fieseler, Dean Karnazes, John Bingham, and Jeff Galloway.

Thank you to Marian and Tom Cooper.

Thank you to the countless clients over the years who have trusted me to guide them through to the finish line of their races.

And thank you to Scott Harrison, Ann Williams, Gina Zangrillo, Beth Martin, Jill Italiano, Susan Tyrrell, Clint Tebbetts, Doug Schwartz, Michael and Michelle Buscher, William Beardsley, Nancy Cronin, Patrick Holden, Lynn DiMenna, Maura Brickman, Suzy McCarthy, Cathy Monahan, Vasso Kelly, Andrew Dover, Kate Harrison, Joe O'Callaghan, Matt Sedgwick, and John Thompson.

ABOUT THE AUTHOR

Tom Holland, M.S., C.S.C.S., is an exercise physiologist with a master's degree in exercise science. He has also been certified by the American College of Sports Medicine, the National Strength and Conditioning Association, the National Academy of Sports Medicine, and the American Council on Exercise.

A sub-three-hour marathoner and eight-time Boston Marathon finisher, Tom has run in more than fifty marathons around the world. He has also completed four ultramarathons, including the JFK fifty-miler in Maryland, and the thirty-six-mile "Run to the Sun," to the 10,028-foot summit of Mount Haleakala on Maui. Tom is a twelve-time Ironman triathlete with finishes in New Zealand, Germany, South Korea, Malaysia, and Australia.

Tom has also starred in numerous fitness videos, including *Tom Holland's Total Body Workout, Tom Holland's Total Ab Workout,* and *The Abs Diet Workout.* He hosts the weekly radio show "Real Fitness" and is the author of *The 12-Week Triathlete.* In 2006, Tom introduced his own line of fitness clothing, TeamHolland Fitness Apparel.

Tom lives in Connecticut with his wife Philippa, his son Tommy, and his black lab Lucy.